THE ART OF SHAVING

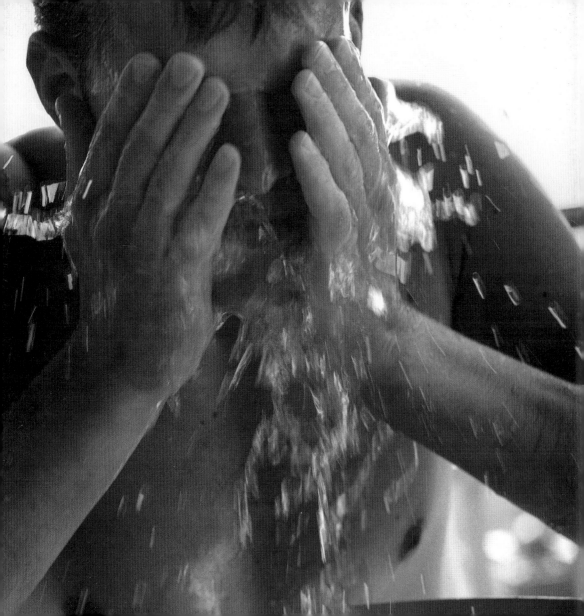

THE **ART**
OF **SHAVING**

MYRIAM ZAOUI
AND **ERIC MALKA**

PHOTOGRAPHS
BY SUSAN SALINGER

CLARKSON POTTER/PUBLISHERS
NEW YORK

Text copyright © 2002 by Eric Malka and Myriam Zaoui
Photographs copyright © 2002 by Susan Salinger

Published by Clarkson Potter/Publishers, New York, New York.
Member of the Crown Publishing Group, a division of Random House, Inc.
www.randomhouse.com

CLARKSON N. POTTER is a trademark and POTTER and colophon are registered trademarks of Random House, Inc.

THE ART OF SHAVING is a registered trademark and tradedress of M.O. Industries, Inc.

Printed in Singapore

Design by Caitlin Daniels Israel

Library of Congress Cataloging-in-Publication Data

Zaoui, Myriam.
    The art of shaving/Myriam Zaoui and Eric Malka; photographs by Susan Salinger.
    Includes index.
    1. Shaving.   I.Malka, Eric.   II. Title.
TT964 .M35 2002
646.7'24—dc21   2001050033

ISBN 0-609-60915-7

10   9   8   7   6

First Edition

CONTENTS

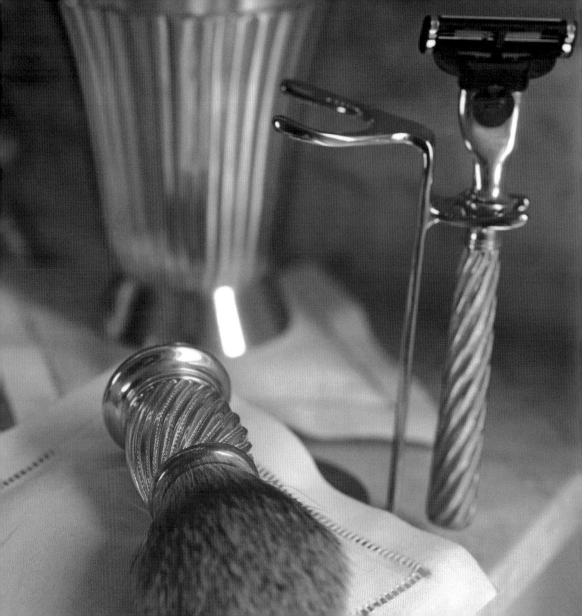

INTRODUCTION

Shaving plays a crucial role in every man's life. It has been considered one of the earliest symbols of upbringing and machismo; it's most definitely *the* fundamental right of passage from boyhood to manhood; and it remains the ever-present reminder that our body and skin are perpetually growing and evolving. In 2000 B.C., as an indication of royalty, metal beards were tied with ribbons or straps to the chins of kings. In 300 B.C., twenty-one-year-old Roman men were given their first ceremonious shave, followed by an elaborate party. And today, nearly every male adolescent—whatever his race, class, or religion—is inducted one way or another into the hall of shaving.

Since the dawn of shaving, men have been in hot pursuit of the perfect shave. In an attempt to achieve optimal results while trying to maximize the comfort factor, manufacturers of shaving products and tools have been striving for the ultimate shaving solution, experimenting with—and developing—new implements to meet men's every grooming need. And to this day, the pursuit is still very much alive.

Over the years we too have been in hot pursuit of the perfect shave, eager to test out new shaving accoutrements to see if they would help alleviate the host of shaving injuries I suffered. One day, as I was walking through the streets of London, I decided to leave my scratchy and poorly shaven face to the hands of a professional barber. Much to my surprise, the results were unlike anything I had ever seen or felt before: my face was smooth and cleanly shaven, my skin felt refreshed, and I had actually enjoyed the whole process. Since that day, I've been a dedicated convert to the art of wet shaving, realizing that the perfect shave is a unique combination of different factors: tools, products, and wet-shaving techniques.

One of my oldest and fondest childhood memories is of watching my father shave in the morning and smelling the soothing scent of his aftershave as he finished his daily ritual. I couldn't wait until I was old enough to grow facial hair of my own and to be able to shave like him. In fact, I was so eager to engage in the practice that one day, when I was about five, I decided to give it a try. My mother, who had just put me in the tub for a bath, briefly walked out of the room to get a towel from the hall closet. As soon as she was out of sight, I leaped out of the water and went straight for my father's safety razor, which was sitting on the edge of the sink, and proudly ran the blade down my cheek. My mother found me, razor in hand, with a huge grin on my face and a sparkle in my eye. Unfortunately, and much to her dismay, I was also covered in blood.

You can still see the scar on my right cheek. Although the experience was certainly indelible, if I were to do it all over again, I would take some advice from the pros first.

The purpose of this book—the result of seven years of professional shaving and skin-care expertise (and a lifetime of shaving)—is to provide you with all the information you'll need to get an ultraclose, smooth, and comfortable shave. First, we'll take you through a brief history of shaving, then discuss the ins and outs of what it takes—and what you'll need—to achieve the ultimate in the art of shaving. Step by step, we'll show you how to select the right shaving tools, how to use and maintain them, how to pick out shaving products that are beneficial to your skin type, and how to cure and help prevent common shaving injuries. We'll teach you the *right* shaving techniques, so you won't be left with a scar under your cheek. And we hope to provide you with all the shaving knowledge you'll ever need to pass on to future generations of shavers.

—ERIC MALKA

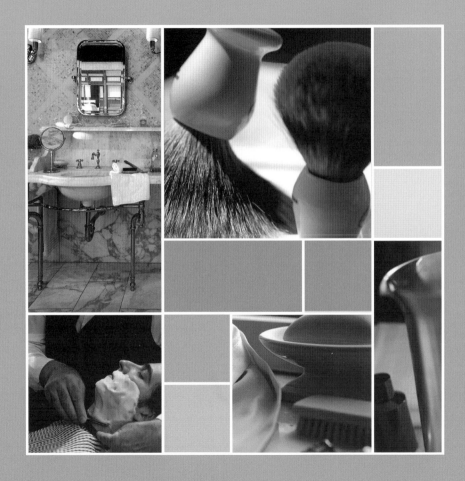

1 THE HISTORY OF SHAVING

SHAVING THROUGH THE CENTURIES

The history of shaving goes back more than a hundred thousand years, when man first started coming up with ways to remove hair from his body, perhaps to differentiate himself from animals. Cave paintings from Neanderthal times show men plucking whiskers with two seashells. A few centuries later, flint—a gray stone that can easily be sharpened but is not very durable—became the tool of choice. It wasn't until about 4000 B.C., however, that the reason for facial-hair removal and grooming—that is, health—became more apparent. The ancient Egyptians were notorious for their quasi-obsession with hygiene and hairless (and lice-free) bodies; visible hair on any part of the body bordered on criminal. Both men and women shaved their heads and sported wigs, and they concocted depilatory creams containing scary ingredients like arsenic and quicklime to help dissolve unsightly hairs.

Egyptian men thought that having facial hair was an indication of poor hygiene, so it was very common for wealthy Egyptians to have a barber on staff. In Mesopotamia, barbers were highly esteemed in society, right up there with dignitaries and doctors. Every town had a street on which barber shops were lined up. For a small fee, Mesopotamians got treated to a shave with a razor and pumice stone, and to a perfumed oil massage afterward.

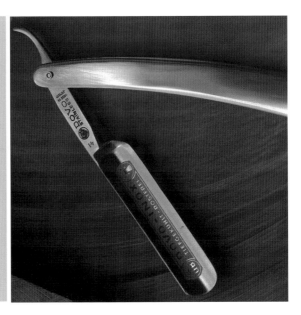

With the advent of metalwork about a century later, shaving tools became more sophisticated and efficient. Sharpened copper-alloy disks and blades, and later bronze and iron ones, provided a closer shave. Pretty soon, Greeks, Romans, and Scandinavians jumped on the band wagon. The average man from India (400 B.C.) shaved his chest and pubic area; Roman legions used pumice stones to sand off their beards (200 B.C.); Britons shaved every part of their bodies except their heads and upper lips (50 B.C.); and thanks to a wealthy Greek businessman responsible for bringing professional barbers from Sicily to Rome (300 B.C.), the professional shave became de rigueur.

From around A.D. 100 to the early seventeenth century, beards came back into fashion. The trend was started by Emperor Hadrian (76–138 A.D.), who grew one to hide his horrendous complexion. But as Louis XIII of France, who occupied the throne in 1610, began to lose his hair, beards again fell out of favor. The next two hundred years saw tremendous advancements in shaving tools. Around 1680, the first straight razor made its appearance in Sheffield, England. A few years later, cast steel—a hard metal able to hold an edge better and longer—was invented, precipitating and no doubt contributing to the writing of Jean-Jacques Perret's famous treatise *"La Pogonotomie"* (The Art of Learning to Shave Oneself). The French cutler proposed the novel idea that men shave themselves, a task that up until then was primarily left to barbers or close relatives.

The middle of the nineteenth century proved to be a big turning point. In 1847, the English inventor

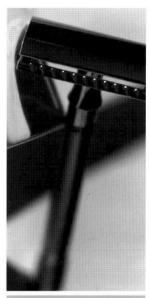

Alexander the Great takes credit for popularizing shaving in Greece. He is said to have ordered his soldiers to shave so that the beard could not be used as a grip to facilitate throat-slashing and decapitation by the enemy.

William Henson designed the first "hoe type" razor, placing the handle perpendicular to the blade, making it easier to grip and control. Overnight, the new razor became a huge success, launching a whole new category of male grooming. Homemade shaving soaps, creams, and lotions were bubbling and being perfected all over England. Meanwhile, in the United States, the Kampfe brothers filed a patent in 1880 for the first "safety razor," with a wire skin guard along one side of the razor's edge that left the other side exposed for shaving. The blade required frequent and arduous sharpening, but it was still the best shave in town.

A few years later, the soon-to-be-famous King Camp Gillette, then a salesman for the Baltimore Seal Company, came up with a razor with a disposable blade, which completely revolutionized shaving. In 1901, he teamed up with engineers from the Massachusetts Institute of Technology to design a disposable double-edged blade set in a T-shaped handle, which enabled the user to open up the top of the razor, remove the dull blade, and replace it. World War I proved to be a huge marketing opportunity for Gillette, when the U.S. Armed Forces turned to him to supply all safety razors and blades for each and every man on his way to Europe. Gillette became a household name.

In 1927, Lieutenant Colonel Jacob Schick invented the first electric dry shaver, a tool that operated on oscillating blades, whose bulky motor was eventually replaced by a power cord and batteries. A decade later, Old Spice—still today's best-selling brand of aftershave—hit the shelves.

The first commercially successful "coated-edge" blade, one covered with polyetrafluoroethylene (abbreviated PTFE) to effectively glide over the face, was introduced by Wilkinson in 1961; and by 1965, the first disposable cartridge razor appeared, complete with blade and separate plastic handle. It didn't need sharpening, maintenance, or even replacing. Economical, simple, and practical: two or three shaves and it was history—in the trash, and out came a new one.

Six years later, Gillette developed the twin-blade razor and cartridge, quickly followed by one set on a pivot so it could adjust to the contours of the face, keeping the blade at the best cutting angle. Shortly after that, the first cheap plastic disposable razor with a blade built into the head was made available.

Today's manufacturers are constantly developing shaving tools and products to further improve results and to render the art of shaving as smooth and as pleasurable as possible. As recently as 2000, the first triple-blade razor—providing three times the cutting power in a single stroke. But as with most practices, the art of shaving is a constantly evolving science, one that is doing so at lightning speed.

THE HISTORY OF BARBERING

There was a time when a gentleman went to the barber for anything from a shave, haircut, and manicure to bloodletting, cauterization, and tonsil and tooth removal. In fact, the barber's dual role of surgeon and groomsman goes back to

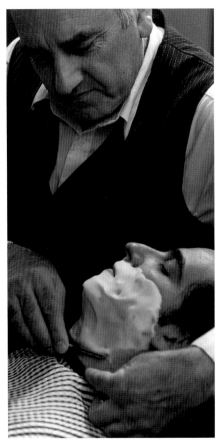

1600 B.C., when the Egyptians used knives to give haircuts and perform surgery. The traditional striped red-and-white barber pole is a symbolic remnant of these times—the two red spiral ribbons represent two long bandages, one twisted around the arm before bleeding and the other for binding it afterward. Fortunately, over the years, the two roles have been separated, and barbering has become a serious and respected art.

Barber comes from *barba,* the Latin word for "beard." The earliest barbers date back to primitive man, who believed that good and bad spirits inhabited the body through hair, and that the only way to get rid of bad spirits was to cut off hair. Consequently, the community barber held one of the most esteemed and privileged positions in society. Over the course of the centuries, however, as shaving evolved into an art that could readily be practiced from home, barbering lost some of its cachet and dignity, only to be relinquished to the backburners of society; the barber sought refuge in the role of wigmaker.

In the late nineteenth century, however, the profession enjoyed a new high when a barber school, the first institution of its kind in the world, opened in Chicago. Its success was apparent from the start, and branches sprang up all over the country. Pretty soon, barbershops were offering unparalleled professional shaving services as well as a place to just "hang out." Today, professional barbers have reignited this age-old practice. In addition to satisfying the trimming, shaving, and cutting needs of contemporary man, their shops have become places where shaving information and tips are readily exchanged. A barbershop offers respite from the daily rituals of everyday life and is an oasis for the well-groomed gentleman.

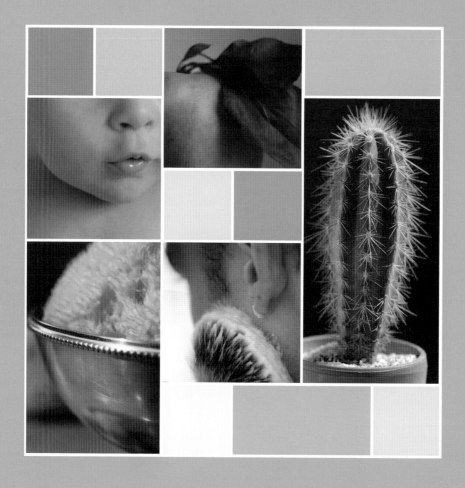

2 THE SKIN OF SHAVING

THE IMPORTANCE OF PROPER SKIN CARE

Proper care and daily maintenance of your skin is one of the best gifts you can give yourself, as well as *the* best way to prepare your skin for a shave. Like every other routine, daily skin care becomes second nature once you've figured out your skin type and how and when to take care of it.

Only in the last few years have men started to take notice of their skin—or, more specifically, the importance of taking care of it on a daily basis. The skin-care industry responded quickly by offering a multitude of products geared toward men. There are products for cleansing, scrubbing, moisturizing, and cell regeneration and tissue growth. You can find something for all skin types: oily, dry, normal, sensitive, aging, and problem. All products on the market contain a variety of ingredients that are important to consider when selecting what works best for you.

WHAT IS SKIN?

Our skin, composed of a number of layers of cells, is a constantly changing organ. From the smooth and supple skin of babyhood to the dry, wrinkled, and coarse skin of maturity, skin accounts for about 20 percent of our body weight and measures about 2.1 square yards for a person of average size. It transports forty-two gallons of blood and one to three gallons of water each day. The skin is the only organ in direct contact with the outside world at all times; it's constantly subjected to external aggressions and everyday stresses, as well as to the body's own internal mechanism. Smoke, pollution, stress, fear, anxiety, age, lack of sleep, lack of fluids, lack of exercise, improper diet, chemicals, alcohol, caf-

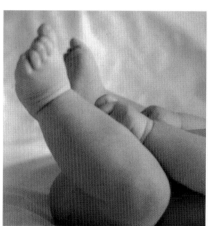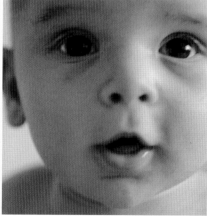

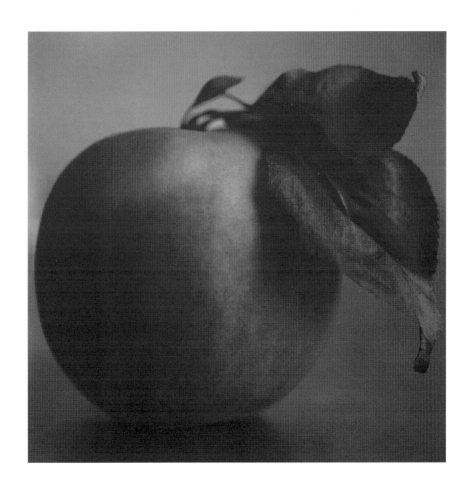

feine, frustration, hormonal changes, toxins, wind, sun, heat, ultraviolet rays, cold, and a host of culprits affect not only how your skin looks and feels but also how quickly it regenerates or ages.

The skin protects the body against the elements and the penetration of dirt, germs, and foreign bodies such as toxins, alkalines, and acids. It regulates the body's temperature through perspiration and through narrowing and expanding blood vessels. It renews itself every month or so, getting rid of a dead coat of cells and replacing it with a new coat. And it even wards off foreign perpetrators by developing its own protective shell, called the acid mantle, which eliminates germs with the help of a host of "beneficial germs" that reside on the skin's surface, as well as through perspiration and secreted carbon dioxide. But the skin remains grossly neglected, often ignored, and usually unrewarded.

The skin on your face and neck, in particular, needs a lot of attention. Unlike the skin elsewhere, it's particularly thin and sensitive and has a high concentration of sebaceous glands, especially around the "T" zone, an area that covers the top of your brow down to your nose and the middle of your chin. And because you'll also be shaving it, facial skin needs even more care.

There are two things you're looking to do for your skin. First, you want to restore and/or maintain a balanced pH level. The skin's pH (or hydrogen-ion concentration) indicates its acidity. A balanced or neutral pH (in the 6.5–7 range) is most beneficial for the skin. If the pH is above 7, then the skin is too alkaline; if it's below 7, it's too acidic. To maintain a neutral pH, you should use shampoos and soaps that have a neutral pH. Second, you want to ensure that the sebaceous glands are producing the right amounts of sebum, a natural skin moisturizer (see sidebar, opposite).

WHAT'S YOUR SKIN TYPE?

People have different types of skin—oily, dry, sensitive, and prematurely aging—caused not only by genetic predisposition but also by everyday stresses, including environmental, physical, and emotional ones.

OILY SKIN

Individuals with oily skin tend to have overactive sebaceous glands that leave too much oil on the skin's surface. The skin takes on a shiny appearance; dilated pores become clogged, causing pimples and blackheads. During the summer months oily skin gets even oilier because the heat and humidity cause blood vessels to dilate and increase perspiration and sebum production.

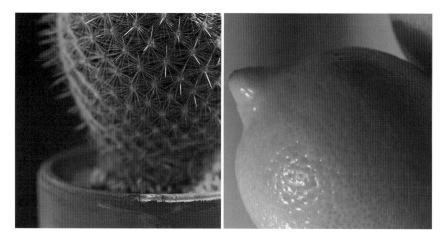

Although it might sound like a contradiction, the best way to treat oily skin is not by drying it out. Using skin-drying alcohol, astringents, and harsh cleansers will cause sebaceous glands to go into overdrive, producing even more sebum to compensate. Too much exfoliating or overscrubbing produces the same result. Instead, we recommend that you use products that contain specific essential oils that help restore and maintain the acid mantle, and gently drain sebum from the glands without stimulating them. Make sure you cleanse your skin thoroughly and regularly with a mild cleanser, morning and night. Follow with a mild alcohol- and oil-free moisturizer. After each shave, apply aftershave gel.

DRY SKIN

Dry skin is caused by insufficient sebum production. As a result, the acid mantle becomes unbalanced, and water has a difficult time penetrating the skin's surface. The skin becomes dehydrated, pores tighten, and especially during cold, dry winter months, blood vessels constrict. Dry skin is also prone to developing wrinkles faster.

If you have dry skin, avoid anything that is an astringent or contains alcohol. The best way to treat dry skin is to replace its lost moisture with moisturizers that are rich in natural vegetable oils (some of which, like hazelnut or almond oil, are naturally cleansing) and essential oils that naturally enhance sebum production (geranium, carrot seed, ylang-ylang, and frankincense). Avoid soaps that can further strip moisture, and keep to a minimum hot facial steam baths that stimulate circulation. We recommend facial gels or fatty liquid soaps. After cleansing, follow up with moisturizer every morning and before bedtime.

SENSITIVE SKIN

Sensitive skin is evidenced by uncomfortable burning, itching, inflammation, redness, allergic reactions, and/or dermatitis. More so than any other skin types, it's particularly reactive to toxins, stress, insufficient exercise and sleep, changing weather conditions, poor diet and health, chemicals, lack of oxygen, dirt, and pollution. It should be treated with mildness and moderation—nothing should be too hot, too oily, too dry, or too harsh. Follow the same facial routine as you would for any other skin type, making sure you use ultramild soaps and hypoal-

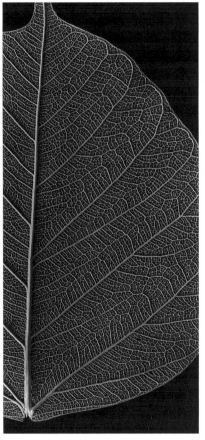

lergenic products that are chemical-, alkaline-, fragrance-, and alcohol-free. After morning and nighttime cleansing, use a soothing and calming moisturizer that contains natural essential oils such as chamomile, lavender, or jasmine.

PREMATURELY AGING SKIN

Characterized by unusual dryness and the appearance of early wrinkles and facial lines, this condition is a result of loss of moisture, poor oxygenation, and advanced collagen depletion, a normal occurrence in aging. It can be caused by excessive stress, alcohol- and nicotine-abuse, poor diet and health, and all of the other physical, emotional, and environmental factors previously mentioned.

The first thing you need to do—in addition to considering a lifestyle change—is to replenish its moisture. This can be done internally by drinking lots of water, and externally by using a high-quality moisturizer and products containing essential oils that are rejuvenating, that stimulate sebaceous and lymph glands, and that activate blood flow for cell oxygenation. (See chart on pages 32–33.) When you cleanse or apply a moisturizer, gently massage the surface of your skin to activate blood circulation and cell regeneration, the keys to young and healthy-looking skin. Use a facial scrub once or twice a week to deep-clean and remove dead cells. And don't forget to use moisturizer at night.

YOUR FACIAL ROUTINE

Although there are different skin types, we recommend the same facial routine for each. The key is to choose products containing essential oils that are beneficial for your skin type (see pages 32–33). Just remember C–S–M–M: Cleanse, Scrub, Mask, Moisturize.

1. CLEANSE

The purpose of cleansing is to strip your skin of all toxins, perspiration, oils, and impurities. It tones the skin by ridding its surface of dead cells, which, when they accumulate, make the skin look dull. Cleansing also activates blood circulation and lymphatic glands and stimulates the skin-renewal process. And when done properly, it deep-cleans pores, eliminating infection-causing bacteria.

Cleanse your skin twice a day: every morning and every night before going to bed. It's especially important to do so right before shaving. Use a mild facial wash or foaming cleanser, and stay away from harsh soaps or those that contain sodium lauryl sulfate and sodium laureth sulfate, ingredients frequently found in all kinds of soaps, including laundry and dishwashing detergents. (These detergents can dry out the skin and hair, upset the skin's pH balance, produce inflammation of the skin, and severely damage eyes. They're also on the FDA's list of suspected carcinogens.) For directions on use, always follow the manufacturer's instructions.

2. SCRUB

A scrub or exfoliant is a deep-pore cleanser and is ideal for all skin types. It unclogs pores, removes toxins, reoxygenates, activates circulation, stimulates the collagen-building process, gets rid of dead cells, and will leave your skin soft and fresh, with a bright-colored complexion. Use it once or twice a week. Do not, however,

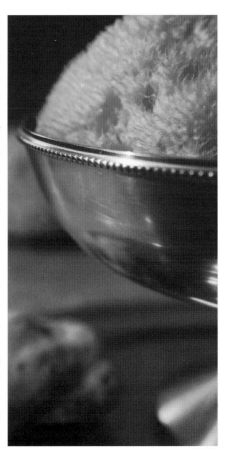

Many cleansing products—including soaps, shampoos, and scrubs—seem to pride themselves on the fact that they provide a lot of suds for "squeaky clean" results. But many also disrupt the skin's natural pH balance, leaving it dry and flaky. Furthermore, if your skin has a tendency to be oily, drying cleansers *worsen* the condition: the skin goes into oil-production overdrive to compensate. The excess production of oil can lead to (or exacerbate) acne. If, on the other hand, your skin is dry, the last thing you want to do is make it even dryer with dehydrating products.

use a scrub right before or after shaving when the skin is either about to have its external layer removed (during shaving) or when it's sensitive as a result of shaving. Give the skin a chance to rejuvenate and heal—twenty-four hours is usually enough—before you scrub. Look for a scrub that has small beads in it; avoid those with a sandlike consistency or large beads, which can be irritating. Always follow the manufacturer's instructions, and focus on the "T" zone, the area prone to developing blackheads and pimples.

3. MASK

There are different types of masks, each addressing different skin concerns. Some masks are meant to replenish the skin's lost nutrients; others to soothe and calm; others to rejuvenate and stimulate, or even to reduce wrinkles. Some are made with clay to soak up toxins and dirt (different-colored clays have different properties) and some contain nourishing essential oils or nutrients and minerals (extracted from plants or the earth). Use a mask once or twice a week, at night when the skin is more receptive to absorbing nutrients. Never use a mask right before shaving, and always follow the manufacturer's instructions.

4. MOISTURIZE

Moisturizing restores the skin's lost moisture and rebalances the condition of the skin, leaving it smooth and firm. Moisturizing also helps regenerate and replenish nutrients and adds a protective layer to help fight off environmental stresses like dirt and pollution. The best time to moisturize is right after cleansing in the morning and at bedtime. Stay away from products that contain mineral oil, petrolatum, propylene glycol, and all petroleum by-products, all of which can clog pores and cause pimples and blackheads. These products also have long-term drying effects that damage and prematurely age the skin.

SELECTING THE RIGHT PRODUCTS

By far, the best skin-care products are those that in the process of cleansing, scrubbing, masking, and moisturizing will also restore a balanced pH level and won't destroy the acid mantle. You'd be surprised at how many products out there wreak havoc on your skin because they contain chemicals, dyes, synthetic perfumes, alcohol, harsh detergents, and so on (see page 34). They cause skin irritations and allergic reactions; they clog pores and affect the acid mantle and sebum production.

We strongly recommend that you look for products containing natural ingredients such as vitamins (vitamin C specifically boosts skin tone), plant and

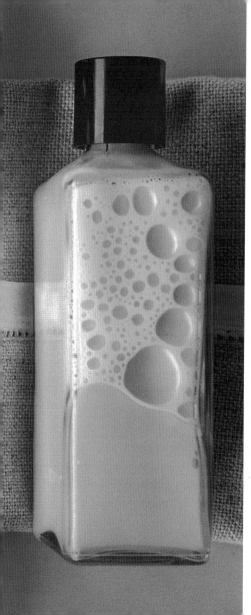

mineral extracts, natural vegetable oils (avocado, almond, jojoba), wax, and natural essential oils. Natural ingredients, unlike their synthetic counterparts, are biodegradable and work in harmony with the body's natural functions and cycles.

The use of essential oils is called aromatherapy, an integral part of the art of shaving. Essential oils are 100 percent natural, concentrated essences of plants, roots, fruits, or flowers. Despite their name, they are not oily, and they evaporate almost immediately upon contact with skin. Essential oils can treat chapped skin, heal blemishes, reduce inflammation, revitalize tired skin, or hydrate surface cells (see pages 32–33). They can be absorbed by the body in several ways: inhaled directly by putting a few drops on a handkerchief or into a diffuser; added to your bathwater; or diluted in vegetable oils that are applied to your skin. Look for premixed products that have a few drops of essential oils blended into an all-natural base.

ESSENTIAL OILS CHART

Oils Categorized by Skin Type	Baby Skin	Blemished Skin	Chapped Skin	Clogged Skin	Dehydrated Skin	Dry Skin	Facial Lines	Flabby Skin	General Skin Care	Hydrated Skin	Inflammed Skin, Chronic	Mature Skin	Mixed Skin	Normal Skin	Oily Skin	Sensitive Skin	Tired Skin	Wrinkled Skin
Anise							■	■										■
Basil				■														
Bergamot									■				■	■	■			
Camphor							■						■					
Cedarwood						■			■	■				■	■			
Chamomile	■					■							■	■			■	
Cypress							■			■		■			■			■
Fennel							■	■				■						■
Geranium					■	■			■			■		■	■			
Immortelle			■															
Jasmine						■			■							■		
Juniper				■											■			
Lavender		■	■			■			■			■	■	■	■			
Lemon		■		■					■						■		■	
Myrrh												■						
Myrtle									■									
Neroli							■		■					■				
Orange	■								■						■	■	■	

Oils Categorized by Skin Type	Baby Skin	Blemished Skin	Chapped Skin	Clogged Skin	Dehydrated Skin	Dry Skin	Facial Lines	Flabby Skin	General Skin Care	Hydrated Skin	Inflammed Skin, Chronic	Mature Skin	Mixed Skin	Normal Skin	Oily Skin	Sensitive Skin	Tired Skin	Wrinkled Skin
Patchouli			■					■		■		■						
Peppermint			■												■			
Rose	■			■	■				■			■		■	■	■		
Rosemary		■													■		■	
Rosewood					■				■					■				
Sage		■						■									■	
Sandlewood			■	■		■			■		■				■			
Tea tree		■																
Thyme		■																
Vetiver													■					
Ylang-ylang					■				■						■			

ESSENTIAL OILS

The practice of using essential oils for medicinal and cosmetic purposes is at least six thousand years old. Throughout the centuries, ancient civilizations have heralded the numerous benefits of these oils. From the Ancient Egyptians to the Greeks, Romans, Arabs, Chinese, and North American Indians, essential oils have been used for their antibacterial and antiseptic properties, incorporated into relaxation techniques, and cherished for their therapeutic characteristics.

INGREDIENTS TO AVOID

Chemical Dyes

FD&C colors, D&C colors, and HC colors are dyes found in many skin-care and shaving products (e.g., green shaving gels, pink soaps, blue shaving foam, etc.). They are harsh chemicals that can cause allergic reactions and rashes, and are a proven carcinogen to laboratory animals.

Synthetic Fragrances

According to the FDA, synthetic or artificial fragrances can cause headaches, allergies, dizziness, skin rashes, skin discoloration and irritation, coughing, and vomiting. Most allergic reactions from cosmetics are caused by their synthetic or artificial fragrances.

Detergents

TEA, DEA MEA, and sodium lauryl sulfate are ingredients added to products to help generate foam and to strip the skin of basically everything on its surface. They are found primarily in soaps, face cleansers, shaving creams, and shampoos, but also in household cleaning products, dishwashing liquids, and toothpaste. They can cause dermatitis, asthma, dry skin, and severe eye damage.

Petroleum and Petroleum By-Products

Petrochemical by-products, such as paraffin, mineral oil, and petrolatum, have an oily or Vaseline-like consistency and are used as cheap substitutes to natural oils that are harmless to the skin but expensive. Petrochemical by-products clog pores and prevent the skin's natural respiration process.

Preservatives and Alchohol

Methyl, propyl, butyl, and imidazolidinyl urea are all preservatives. According to the FDA, the second most leading cause of allergic skin reactions (after synthetic dyes) are artificial preservatives.

Any product name that finishes with "ol" is an alcohol or alcohol-derivative. And anything that contains alcohol can cause skin dryness, peeling, burning, swelling, and skin eruptions.

Now that you've learned the ins and outs of skin care and the importance of maintaining a skin-care routine on a daily basis, you'll quickly reap the benefits. In a matter of days, you'll begin to notice a change in skin tone, texture, and probably color. Your friends might even comment on your new glow and suspect a new love in your life. Just leave them guessing.

AROMATHERAPY

Like our bodies, skin needs nourishment on a regular basis. The best way to provide nourishment to the skin is through aromatherapy, or the use of pure essential oils. These oils possess many different therapeutic properties, and they're naturally hydrating and rich in nutrients. Made from very small molecules that penetrate the layers of the skin, they promote cell rejuvenation, improve blood circulation, and strengthen the connective tissue, thereby reducing the appearance of wrinkles. Essential oils are immediately absorbed by the skin's surface and do not leave any oily residue whatsoever.

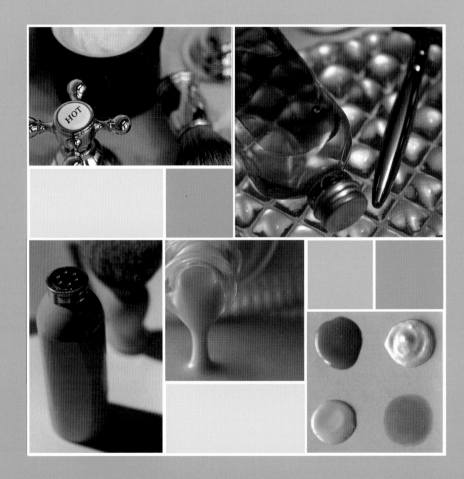

3 THE PRODUCTS OF SHAVING

It's not enough simply to have the right shaving tools and to know how to use and care for them. Selecting the right products is just as important to the art of shaving. They can also make the difference between healthy skin and skin that's irritated by ingrown hairs, razor burn, and nicks and cuts.

There are many products on the market, available in different forms and packages, serving different purposes. They include preshaves, shaving soaps, creams, oils, foams, gels, depilatories, and, of course, aftershaves; and they come in all sorts of shapes and sizes, including bottles, tubes, jars, cans, tubs, and even bowls. But before selecting which products work best for you, it's important to familiarize yourself with what they do, how they're used, when to use them, what ingredients to look for, and which ones to stay away from. We recommend that you avoid shaving products that contain synthetic fragrances, dyes, and alcohol, all of which can cause skin irritations, redness, and dryness. Instead, select those that contain only natural ingredients, such as essential oils, algae, and vegetable oils.

PRESHAVE CARE AND PRODUCTS

After you've thoroughly prepared your skin for the shave (see page 75), it's time for the first step: preshave care. This is one of the most important factors in the art of wet shaving, but also one that's often neglected. The purpose of preshave products is twofold: they add a protective layer to the skin that serves as a buffer between the sharpness of the blade and the sensitivity of the skin; and they warm the skin to open pores and soften the beard. In addition, the mere process of applying the product massages the skin, stimulates blood flow, and lifts the beard off the face.

PRESHAVE OILS

Properties: Protects the Skin
The preshave product we recommend the most—especially for men with ingrown hairs, razor burn, or sensitive skin—is preshave oil. It provides the maximum amount of protection; your blade glides on the surface of your face to catch the hairs but not the skin itself. And preshave oils *do not* leave an oily residue on the skin after shaving: the oil simply rests on the surface of the skin during the shave and is wiped off clean during the shaving process.

Make sure you select a preshave oil that contains natural oils, such as vegetable or castor oil. In addition to being biodegradable, natural oils are

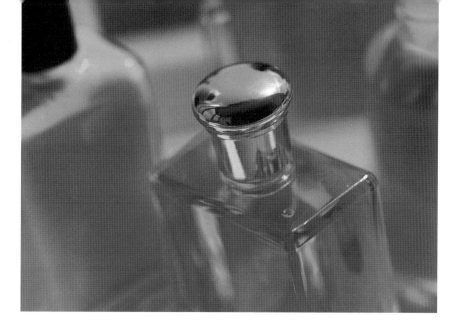

healthier. And because they're made up of larger molecules, they remain on the skin's surface without penetrating the pores. Avoid preshave oils that contain synthetic or chemical oils (such as mineral oil and petrolatum, both petrochemical by-products), which can clog pores, prevent the skin's natural respiration, and cause pimples and blackheads. And always stay away from anything that contains alcohol or alcohol by-products, such as those that end in "ol," like propylene glycol.

Properties: Softens the Beard

Preshave oil makes the whiskers more pliable for the shave, a crucial step in wet shaving. We highly recommend oils that contain clove, black pepper, or sandalwood essential oils, all of which are readily absorbed by the beard and are naturally warming, which further opens pores and softens the beard. Avoid ingredients such as peppermint, camphor, eucalyptus, and rosemary, whose cooling effect causes pores to tighten and whiskers to stiffen.

Use

A nickel-size drop of preshave oil will do the trick. Rub it in the palm of your hands and massage it into your beard. Finish massaging with an upward motion to lift the beard off the face. Remember to thoroughly wash your hands with soap and water to avoid getting slippery oil on your tools.

Crucial to shaving and to obtaining optimal results, the preparation for the shave contributes immensely to the comfort, safety, and speed of the actual shaving process. In addition to providing adequate hydration to the whiskers, proper preparation lubricates the skin so that the blade can glide smoothly over the face, minimizing the chances of nicks, cuts, razor burn, and skin irritations.

PRESHAVE GELS

Properties

Preshave gel is similar to oil in that its purpose is to lubricate. Some men prefer gel because it doesn't make your hands as oily. However, we don't recommend gel because, unlike oil, it doesn't provide adequate protection: gels are usually water-soluble, so they blend right into the shaving cream instead of resting on your skin's surface.

Use

Apply preshave gel as you would preshave oil: squeeze a small amount into your palm, rub your palms together, and massage the gel into your beard. Finish massaging with an upward motion to lift the beard off the face as much as possible. Wash and rinse hands after use.

PRESHAVE SCRUBS

Properties

Preshave scrubs' or exfoliants' purpose is to deep-cleanse pores, to buff skin, and to remove the external layer or dead skin cells. Although scrubs are often marketed as shaving products, they're actually more about skin care. We don't advise using a scrub or exfoliant before shaving. During the shaving process itself, you're already removing a layer of skin with the razor's blade. This is precisely the reason why you need to *add* a protective layer to your skin before shaving (the purpose of the preshave oil). If you use a scrub before shaving, you're removing a layer of skin before you even get to the shaving part! And the more layers you remove, the more sensitive your skin will be, and the more susceptible you'll be to razor burn.

Use

So if you're going to use a scrub, do it in a timely fashion, either right before going to bed or on a day when you know you won't be shaving. You need to give the outer layer of skin plenty of time to regenerate before taking the blade to it. Use the scrub once or twice a week, and focus on the "T" zone: the area that extends from your forehead, right above your eyebrows, down to your nose and the middle of your chin. The "T" zone is prone to excess oil because of the large number of oil-producing sebaceous glands right underneath the skin's surface in that particular area, so it's a favorite spot for blackheads and pimples. Thoroughly wash your face with soap and water beforehand, because you don't want to be rubbing extra dirt and oil into your skin while you're exfoliating.

PRODUCTS FOR THE ACTUAL SHAVE

These shaving products—what you apply to your face before you run the razor over it—are broken down into several categories: shaving creams (lathering and nonlathering), soaps, oils, gels and foams, and depilatories. Some you apply with a shaving brush, some with your fingers, and others with either one.

SHAVING CREAMS

The Lather-up Shaving Cream

Properties

This is by far the best and most effective product for the wet shave. It generates the richest possible lather; protects and lubricates your skin, leaving it smooth and moisturized; and lifts whiskers off the face. The cream is applied with either a badger-hair shaving brush or your fingers, but we recommend a brush: the bristles have the added advantages of generating a warm lather, of further lifting the beard off your face, and of gently exfoliating the skin.

Lather-up creams are sold in jars or tubs, or in small tubes for traveling convenience. They contain between 30 and 50 percent fat (usually coconut oil, an all-natural oil that does not penetrate the skin), as well as glycerin, which is why their lather is so rich and thick, providing the best possible protection. Glycerin, derived from vegetable oil, is important because it serves as a humectant, which locks in water and hydrates the skin. It's also an efficient emollient because it softens the beard and leaves the skin smooth and moisturized. The fat content is essential because it provides the necessary lubrication and protection for the skin during the shaving process, so that the blade just glides over the surface of the skin without irritating or nicking it.

Use

Unlike shaving soaps, creams generate lather quickly. The lather is generated directly on the face, instead of in a bowl or mug. To use, wet your fingers and face or the brush's bristles with hot water. Then dip your fingers into the jar to

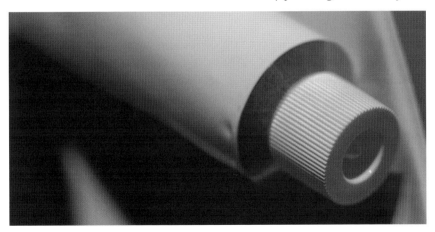

apply the cream directly on your face, or to the center of the brush's tip. Since the cream is concentrated, two fingertips' worth will do the trick. Next, lather up the cream on your face with circular motions using your fingers or a shaving brush. If you use a brush, the cream will last you about twice as long as if you use it with your fingers.

The Nonlathering Shaving Cream

Properties

It's not meant to lather up, and it's applied directly to a wet or dry face with fingers, not with a brush; it has a toothpaste-like consistency. Although some shavers might consider it more convenient because it's faster, the nonlathering cream isn't as effective as the lathering kind. First, because the cream is applied with your fingers, the beard is flattened on your face, making it more difficult for the blade to catch hairs. Second, because you're not using water, your skin is dry and deprived of the necessary moisture. Third, nonlathering creams often contain menthol and benzocaine, a numbing agent, which desensitizes the skin. When your skin is desensitized, it's difficult to monitor the amount of blade pressure you apply because you don't feel as much. So it's easier to get nicks, cuts, or razor burn—you could be cutting yourself and not even noticing it. And finally, the cream is so thick that it clogs the blades. That means you'll

HUMECTANTS

Humectants help prevent excess water loss by evaporation. Some also act as lubricants, others help soften the hair. The most popular humectant used today is glycerin, but sorbitol and mannitol are used to some extent as well.

have to repeatedly rinse the razor between strokes and repeatedly tap it on the edge of the sink to free up the blade.

SHAVING SOAPS

Properties

They made their first appearance in the fourteenth century and were extremely popular until World War I, when lathering and nonlathering shaving creams became widely available. Shaving soaps are similar to lathering creams in terms of results and are popular with shavers who savor the traditional aspect of the shaving experience. A good-quality shaving soap contains a high level of fat (vegetable or tallow) and glycerin to contribute to the richness of the lather, to provide lubrication, and to leave the skin smooth and moisturized. Look for a soap that has a high fat content (30 to 50 percent) and avoid inexpensive shaving soaps, which are often bath or shower soaps in disguise. They don't provide any protection during the shave and can leave skin dry and irritated.

Use

The traditional shaving soap is lathered up with a shaving brush in a container—a mug, bowl, or deep dish. First, wet your brush under running hot water, or fill up your sink with hot water. Don't tap excess water off the brush, because the point is to retain the moisture in the brush so that it gets directly to your face to soften your beard and open the pores. Lather up the soap using circular motions directly in the bowl. At first, the bubbles will appear large, but as you keep going, they'll increase in number and get smaller and smaller until

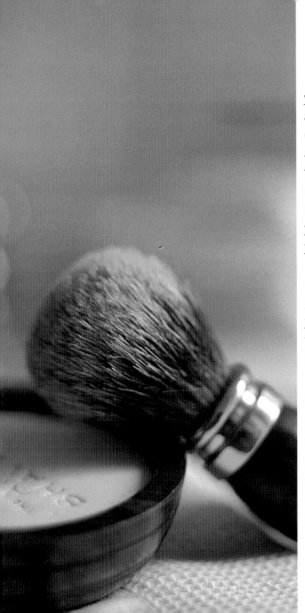

you can barely see them. Once you've achieved a thick and warm lather (which usually takes fifteen seconds), apply it directly to your face with the brush. Continue using circular motions on your face to further increase the lather's density, to soften your beard, and to lift the hairs off your skin.

Unlike lathering creams, traditional soaps require a little more elbow grease to generate lather. The longer you whisk, the richer the lather, and the more your skin will be protected and your shave comfortable.

SHAVING OILS

Properties

The shaving oil is a relatively recent product that first became available in the early 1990s. While it does yield a close shave, it's an uncomfortable one because the oil provides minimal protection for the skin. And shaving oils sometimes contain numbing agents such as menthol or benzocaine, which, as mentioned above, make the skin more prone to nicks, cuts, and razor burn. So if you use shaving oil, be very careful.

Use

The oil is thin and light, and just a few drops are gently massaged onto your wet face right before shaving. The oil spreads easily on the skin and is economical because so little is needed.

SHAVING GELS AND FOAMS

Properties

Foams made their first appearance in 1941 and immediately became popular because they provided fast, easy access to lather with a mere press of a button. The popularity of foams greatly affected the market for creams, which became harder to find, available primarily at specialty shops and high-end drugstores. Gels and foams are popular today not because they're any good, but simply because they're easy to use and easiest to find. But the truth is, they can be quite damaging to your skin.

Many gels and foams contain synthetic perfumes. According to the FDA, synthetic perfumes are the number one cause of skin irritations. They also contain artificial colors and dyes, preservatives, and alcohol, all of which irritate and dry out the skin. They have little oil or lubricants for protection, which makes the shave very uncomfortable and leaves the skin susceptible to razor burn. And as with nonlathering creams and shaving oils, they contain numbing agents that promote cuts, nicks, and irritations. Foams and gels also contain highly toxic and unhealthy gases, such as isobutane and propane, which is what makes them foam in the first place. And the foam that comes out of a can is deceptively rich. It might *appear* rich, but in fact it contains lots of gas and provides very little protection for the skin. In addition, the toxic propellants from the can and gel generate a cold lather, which closes the pores and stiffens the beard (rendering it less manageable), making for a truly uncomfortable shave.

Use

Nevertheless, if you find it absolutely necessary due to circumstances beyond your control to use a foam or a gel—you're in an airport and don't have your shaving gear on hand, or you're in a remote part of the world and it's the only thing available—make sure you apply it to a well-prepared and wet face. To use, apply the foam directly to your wet face, or dispense a small amount of gel into your palm, mix it with water, and apply it to your face.

DEPILATORY CREAMS AND POWDERS

Properties

Depilatory creams and powders don't require the use of a blade, so men who think that razor blades are the number one cause for ingrown hair and razor burn often use them. They're wrong. A blade, when used properly, is *not* the cause of these types of injuries. And in fact depilatory users are exposing themselves to great harm without realizing it.

Here's how they work: depilatories are applied directly to the face, left on for a few minutes, then wiped off with a spatula. They dissolve the hair with calcium thioglycolate, an extremely powerful acid. Putting acid on your skin doesn't make sense. In addition to emitting a highly toxic and unpleasant smell, these products can cause severe skin injuries, including burns, rashes, and irritations, that can result in permanent scarring and skin discoloration. Depilatory creams and powders (the powders are mixed with water to create a paste) are *extremely* dangerous, and you should avoid them at all cost.

Use
Under no circumstances.

AFTERSHAVE CARE AND PRODUCTS

AFTERSHAVES

Properties
Aftershaves were first introduced in barbershops. Barbers used the high-alcohol splashes as antiseptics (they contain as much as 90 percent alcohol) to kill off bacteria and to minimize the transmission of disease from one client to another through shaving instruments; they would also reduce the risk of infection on the client's face; and they smelled nice.

Splashing on aftershave soon evolved beyond its practical purpose and became a tradition, one that our fathers and grandfathers readily picked up. They liked the seemingly revitalizing sensation caused by the alcohol, and the tingling effect. The high alcohol content of these aftershaves, however, left the skin very dry and irritated. In some cases, the tightness and dryness of the skin created a barrier-like surface that was difficult for hairs to pierce through and ingrown hairs developed. The irritated skin often didn't have time to regenerate itself between shaves, making the next shave very uncomfortable. It wasn't until the late 1980s that men started to become more aware of the importance of skin care and its daily maintenance; so a new wave of aftershave products with more beneficial properties was launched.

Aftershaves come in three forms—balms (sometimes called creams), gels, and lotions. They're all really more about skin care and maintenance than anything else. In addition to having antiseptic properties, their purpose is to soothe, moisturize, and regenerate the skin after shaving. Unlike other products used during the actual shave, aftershaves have a longer-lasting effect because they're not immediately wiped off (as shaving cream is).

Some aftershaves are scented; some contain herbal extracts and essential oils; some have a high alcohol content; and some have oil. Others don't have any of these ingredients. Which aftershave you should choose depends on what best suits your skin. (See "The Skin of Shaving," page 19.) An aftershave can soothe, nourish, and moisturize the skin; stimulate cell regeneration; and help maintain clean, healthy skin. Always check product labels carefully, look for all-natural ingredients, and stay away from dyes and synthetic fragrances. It's also a good idea to test the aftershave on your hand (if not on your face) before purchasing it so you can see how it feels on your skin. Make sure the aftershave penetrates your skin without leaving any oily residue.

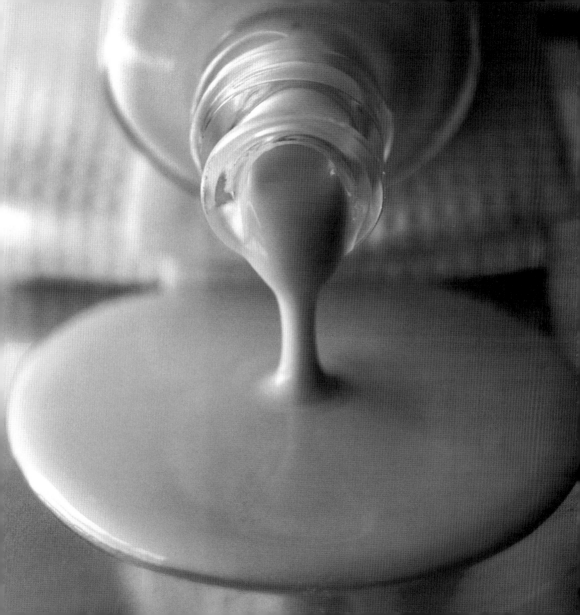

Pat, don't rub, all over your face and neck. Allow to air-dry.

AFTERSHAVE BALMS (CREAMS)

Properties

Although they might be marketed as shaving products, balms are really skin-care products. Many balms contain alcohol (2 to 5 percent), but we think the best ones contain none at all. Alcohol-free balms substitute natural ingredients such as red algae and/or essential oils for alcohol; they are equally antiseptic but don't cause dryness. Because balms contain very little or no alcohol, they're not as dehydrating as splashes and lotions. Balms are recommended for men with sensitive or dry skin, and for use during dry winter months, when there is less moisture in the air and when the skin is prone to dryness. Balms also contain water and oils to moisturize the skin without leaving an oily residue.

Look for balms that contain shea butter (an anti-inflammatory) or natural oils such as grape seed, macadamia, almond, olive, or jojoba, which all have healing and moisturizing properties. Avoid balms that contain nonvegetable or synthetic oils, such as mineral oil or petroleum by-products; these can clog pores and cause pimples. Also, stay away from those that contain alpha-hydroxy acids and salicylic acid; these acids peel off the surface of the skin, causing redness, burning, and rashes. And the last thing you want to do after having removed one layer of skin is to remove another. Finally, avoid balms that contain synthetic fragrances and dyes, which can trigger allergic reactions and cause irritations and burning. It's better to use an unscented aftershave or one that's scented with natural essential oils that don't cause skin irritations. If you want your favorite cologne scent, just dab it on afterward on your shoulders, lower neck, or back of neck. We also recommend that you use balm to relieve or avoid ingrown hairs (see "The Injuries of Shaving," page 97).

Use
Apply the balm all over your face and neck after shaving or at bedtime.

AFTERSHAVE GELS

Properties
Like balms, gels are about skin care. And like balms, they have a fairly low alcohol content compared with lotions—some don't contain any alcohol at all, which is what we prefer. Unlike balms, however, they don't contain oil, which makes them less moisturizing. We recommend balms to men with normal to oily skin, or for use in humid climates. Gels are refreshing and soothing, and they help protect and maintain healthy skin.

Look for gels with natural ingredients such as plant extracts and essential oils for their healing and soothing properties. Some gels contain aloe vera for its astringent, antiseptic, and healing properties. (But try to avoid aloe if you have ingrown hairs or sensitive skin. It will simply aggravate the problem.) We also highly recommend any gel that contains red algae, a natural antiseptic with anti-inflammatory and skin-regenerating properties.

Use
Apply the aftershave gel to the face and neck after shaving (of course).

AFTERSHAVE LOTIONS

Properties

You should use lotions if you're into pain. Of all the aftershaves, lotions have the highest alcohol content (60 to 75 percent) and are very similar to the splashes barbers used in the old days. And you know what happens when you put alcohol on sensitive skin that has just been shaved. *Ouch!* While it's true that alcohol is an antiseptic, we don't recommend using lotions at all because they dry out and irritate the skin, causing redness and burning. In fact, they do absolutely nothing for the skin and don't have any beneficial properties. Also, the alcohol in them drastically tightens the pores. When pores are tight, hairs tend to get caught in them, which can lead to ingrown hairs. And all lotions contain synthetic fragrances and sometimes dyes, which are responsible for most skin irritations and allergic reactions. Stick to balms or gels for the best results.

Use

Don't.

ALUM BLOCKS AND STYPTIC PENCILS

Properties and Use

If you have the misfortune of nicking or cutting yourself—it can happen even in the best of all possible worlds—it's important to treat the wound as quickly as possible and to stop the bleeding before applying any aftershave. Both alum blocks and styptic pencils contain mineral salts that were used by the Egyptians more than four thousand years ago for their healing and antiseptic properties. These salts also help stop bleeding by constricting blood vessels and tightening pores. However, because the minerals are astringent (they pull moisture out of the skin), we don't recommend them to men with dry or sensitive skin.

An alum block is a crystal-like stone that is moistened with cold water and gently rubbed over the entire face, not just on one specific area like a styptic pencil, serving as an antiseptic for razor burn. It helps stop bleeding of nicks and cuts. Because it's larger than a styptic pencil it lasts longer. After use, it should be thoroughly cleaned with water, dried, and stored in a dry place, such as a box. If the stone is wet or exposed to moisture for an extended period of time, it will simply dissolve. Men who use an electric razor often rub alum block all over their faces with warm water to tighten their beards and to raise their whiskers before shaving. The alum block, however, should *never* be used before a wet shave—only after, if necessary.

Unlike the alum block, the styptic pencil is specifically used for individual cuts and nicks. It's derived from the alum block crystal, and its powdered form is concentrated into a stick. Simply moisten the tip of the pencil with water and apply it directly to the nick or cut for a few seconds. It serves as an antiseptic and helps stop the bleeding. The styptic pencil's protective cap and packaging are very convenient for traveling.

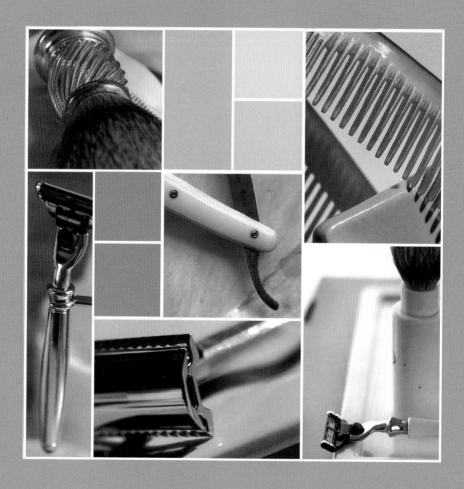

4 THE TOOLS OF SHAVING

We've come a long way since the Stone Age, when men used clamshells, shark teeth ground to a fine edge, or sharpened flint and crude tweezers to remove facial hair. We've evolved considerably since the time when a burning twig with which to singe whiskers was the shaving tool of choice. In fact, from the beginning of shaving history, men have strived to create tools that offer the closest and most comfortable shave. Fortunately, today there's a wide range of safe and efficient shaving instruments: mirrors, cartridge razors, safety razors, straight razors, electric razors, shaving brushes. Some are disposable; some are single-edged, others double- or even triple-edged; some swivel, others are fixed; some you use with water and cream. The choice all depends on what you're looking for, what your preferences are, what's available in your neck of the woods, and how much you're willing to spend.

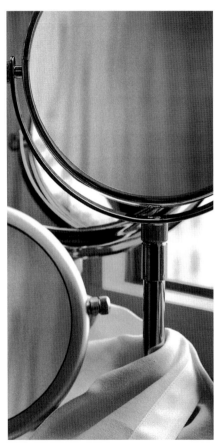

SHAVING MIRRORS

For some, the shaving mirror is the ultimate object of vanity; for others, it's a pathway to the soul. But a mirror is an absolute necessity to study the angles of your face, to monitor your strokes, and to pay attention to detail. Since men first started to use their reflections in water, mirrors have evolved from reflective polished disks of silver, tin, cooper, or bronze (from Greco-Roman times) to sophisticated mirrors—some even fogless—with different magnification.

The two options are fogless and nonfogless (or just plain old) mirrors, each with varying degrees of quality and price. Since many men prefer to shave in the shower, mirrors that won't fog up are popular. They usually come with a suction-cup attachment that adheres to tiles. Be forewarned, however: suction cups sometimes slip, which will cause the mirror to break. And fogless mirrors are not mirrors at all. Unlike real mirrors, which are made from glass and metal, fogless ones are made from bent plastic, and so they tend to scratch and are of lesser quality. You may have to replace your fogless mirror every few months.

Men who shave outside the shower use nonfogless, or regular, mirrors made of glass. There are two basic styles: the standard bathroom mirror attached to the wall or medicine cabinet, and the mirror on a stand. Stand-up mirrors come with different magnification powers: we recommend a magnification of three (three times larger than life); beyond that is too much detail which will obstruct the big picture. The one inconvenience with regular mirrors is that they tend to fog up when in contact with steam and/or hot water. Here's a solution: first, lather up some bath soap in your hands and apply the lather to the face of the mirror. Let the lather sit for about five seconds, then splash hot water on the glass to remove all the soap (don't use your hands or a towel). The mirror will stay fogless for about ten minutes, more than enough time for a shave. Always remember to secure your mirror properly and in a safe place to avoid the chance of its falling and shattering.

RAZORS

CARTRIDGE RAZORS

There are two types, swivel heads and fixed heads. Both have disposable blades, which makes maintenance a cinch.

Swivel-Head Razors

Swivel-head razors were introduced by Gillette in 1971. They are now available to the shaving market with two or three blades (debuted in 2000) and are the most popular of all. On the cutting edge of technology, they not only provide comfort, closeness, and convenience but also can be purchased almost anywhere. There are two types of swivel-head razors: the nondisposable kind, for which you toss the disposable blade and replace it with a new one on a handle that you keep, and the disposable kind, for which you throw away both the blade and the handle once the blade is too dull. The difference in their price—the disposable kind is cheaper—is reflected in their results.

Atra, introduced in 1977, was the first twin-blade shaving system with a pivoting head. Introduced in 1990, Sensor was the first razor with twin blades individually mounted on highly responsive springs that continuously adjust to the face. MACH3, introduced in 1998, was the most significant men's shaving advance since the launch of Gillette's Trac II twin-blade razor. With its three progressively aligned thin, spring-mounted blades and forward pivot action, men can achieve a closer shave in fewer strokes with less irritation.

Swivel heads have the distinct advantage of comfort, closeness, and ease. The blades and head are designed in such a way that they contour every curve on your face, thus greatly decreasing the chances of getting razor burn, nicks, and cuts. Unlike straight razors, the blade never needs to be sharpened. Simply replace it as soon as it's dull, which is usually anytime between three and five shaves, depending on the quality of the blade and the length and thickness of

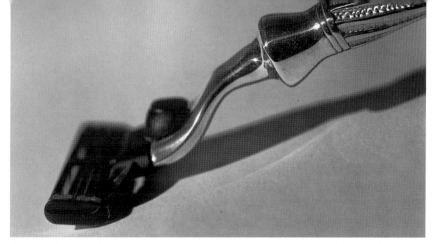

the beard. Basically, when you start feeling resistance on your beard, it's time to switch blades. Some swivel heads even have blades that are mounted on tiny springs to offer still more flexibility. The flexible blades automatically curve inward when too much pressure is applied on the handle while shaving, thus greatly minimizing the possibility of razor burn and serious discomfort.

Nondisposable swivel-head razors are by far the best. Unlike disposable razors that often have a light handle, nondisposable razors have handles with greater heft for more balance, grip, and control—like the difference between writing with a disposable ballpoint or a luxurious fountain pen. The handle itself—not just the blade—plays an important role. If a razor is too light, you'll have a tendency to apply more pressure on the face than is necessary, thus causing razor burn. If the razor is improperly balanced, you're likely to lose control of the handle, increasing the risk of nicks and cuts when it slips. A sturdy, well-balanced razor facilitates the ease with which the blade glides over the face, yielding an even and consistent stroke.

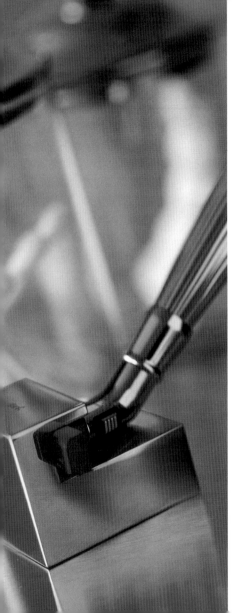

Look for a handle that feels comfortable and solid, and that has a grip that doesn't slip. Look for materials that not only are easy to clean and maintain but also withstand water abuse—sterling silver, buffalo horn, acrylic, or burrthuya wood (a wood found in India that naturally repels water), make ideal handles; they can be easily cleaned with soap and water, then dried with a soft cloth. And also look for handles that are compatible with Gillette MACH3 and Sensor blades, which we think are the best available blades on the market today. They are made of superior quality steel and are very sharp.

Always store the handle and blade away from water. In fact, we recommend storing the razor on a stand in between use. The stand keeps the handle and blade clean and dry, away from bacteria and moisture.

Fixed-Head Razors

Today, almost all fixed-head razors are disposable. They're inexpensive—as low as fifteen cents per razor, as opposed to two dollars for a three-blade disposable swivel. But they're also uncomfortable to shave with because they're so stiff, because

TWIN BLADES

In 1971, Gillette introduced the first twin-blade razor, Gillette Trac II, with two parallel blade edges housed in a single cartridge. Its development was driven by Gillette's earlier discovery of the "hysteresis effect"—the fact that when a blade engages a whisker, it extends the whisker in the hair follicle before cutting it. If a second blade is added to the first, and positioned so that it cuts the hair at the precise moment before retraction, a closer shave results.

they're usually available in a single-blade system only, and because they're made of low-quality steel. When the blade is of poor quality, there is increased resistance between the blade and the hair, making the shave very uncomfortable. Furthermore, the rigid blade doesn't give at all, making it very difficult to contour the curves of the face, which can always lead to nicks or cuts.

SAFETY RAZORS

In 1880, the Kampfe brothers invented a razor called the safety razor. This was a step above the straight or "cut-throat" razor (see "Straight Razors," page 65) because the blade didn't need to be sharpened before each use. King Gillette further revolutionized the concept by inventing a disposable blade at an affordable price, making sharpening completely obsolete. And this was the first T-shaped razor, with a handle to guide the head. Over the years, however, the safety razor has lost a lot of its popularity to the cartridge razor. Fewer and fewer manufacturers make safety razors, even though their blades continue to be sold in most drugstores and supermarkets.

Although considered to be a safer alternative at the time of its invention, by modern standards, *safe* is no longer the first word that comes to mind when describing the razor, especially when compared with the swivel-head cartridge razor. Nevertheless, men who use safety razors swear by them. The classic and traditional appeal of the razor certainly has a few shavers hooked.

Safety razors come in several different models. The basic kind, which is usually the least expensive, features a blade enclosed in a case that can be unscrewed from the handle when it needs replacing. The adjustable safety razor enables the user to select one of five blade positions, depending on the length and thickness of his beard. The mustache razor—a narrower and smaller version of the basic safety razor—has one side smaller than the other. The large

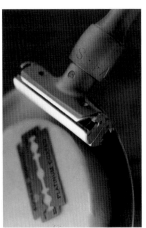

side is for shaping mustaches, goatees, and beards; the smaller side is for hard-to-reach places, like under the nose and around the lips.

Like the cartridge razor, the safety razor needs a good, well-balanced, and comfortable handle. Without one, the razor can slip, increasing the risk of nicks and cuts. If the handle is light, you may apply too much pressure on your face, resulting in razor burn. Look for a handle with a solid, nonslippery grip that sits comfortably in your hand. It should be made from a high-quality material that doesn't rust or tarnish, like nickel or gold-plated

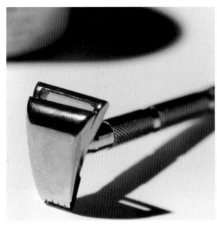

steel. We also recommend that you store your razor on a stand to keep the handle and blade in a clean and dry place, away from bacteria and moisture.

Try to get blades made in Solingen, Germany. They're usually of high quality, made from stainless steel with platinum-coated edges for longer durability and sharpness. Always make sure the blade is clean and dry after each use, and replace it at the first signs of dullness or discomfort. If you're using a safety razor for the first time, use small strokes, starting with the flat areas on your face, then move on to the curves. And remember, practice makes perfect. . . .

STRAIGHT RAZORS

Straight razors—also known as "open razors" or "cut-throats" or "barbershop razors"—were the very first razors available (after sharpened shark teeth and clamshells, of course), first manufactured in Sheffield, England, around 1680. Although they're called razors, they're actually more like knives. Straight razors are available in two types: ones with a permanent blade that needs to be maintained and resharpened, and ones with a disposable blade. Either way, using a straight razor is no easy task. Most of the men who use them today do so out of tradition and hobby. If you decide to use a straight razor for whatever reason, we recommend that you invest some serious time and effort in learning how to use one from a professional barber. Take lessons. Lots of them. You can achieve great results with this art, if the method is correct.

The edge of the straight razor is extremely thin, making it very sharp. After each shave, small grooves are etched into the edge of the blade from cutting whiskers. The grooves make the blade less sharp. Also, as a result of the pressure of the blade on your face, the blade starts to bend back onto itself. The curve in the edge renders the blade less efficient because it's no longer at the optimal angle for cutting. The blade, when not disposable, therefore requires a lot of maintenance to retain its thinness and sharpness.

Taking care of a nondisposable straight

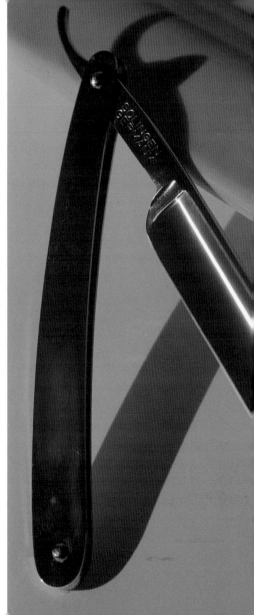

razor blade involves the use of a strop and strop paste. The strop is a beltlike piece that has canvas on one side and leather on the other. Use the canvas side to warm up the blade so that you can "restructure" its edge. Stroke the blade about fifteen times on the canvas side to warm it up, then stroke it about fifteen more on the leather side to smooth out its edge and to reshape it. You need to do this before you use your razor for *each and every shave*. The strop paste is for conditioning and protecting the leather side of the strop, and to help the blade glide over it. Once in a while—perhaps twice a month—condition the leather with paste just before you're about to use the strop. If the razor looses its edge from repeated use and sharpening, you can hone it back to a fine edge on a sharpening stone; this is best done by a professional.

ELECTRIC RAZORS

While we're not proponents of dry shaving, a shaving book wouldn't be complete unless it mentioned electric razors. The concept of a powered razor was unknown until the 1920s, when it was invented by Jacob Schick. The obvious advantage of the new product was that it dispensed with the need for water and cream, enabling the user to shave anywhere within reach of an electrical outlet. In the late 1940s and 1950s, the electric razor was perfected to a self-contained entity in which the motor could run on a large D-size battery. In 1960, Remington introduced the first rechargeable electric razor, making it possible to shave pretty much anywhere, without electricity.

Today, there are two types of dry electric razors: the foil head and the rotary

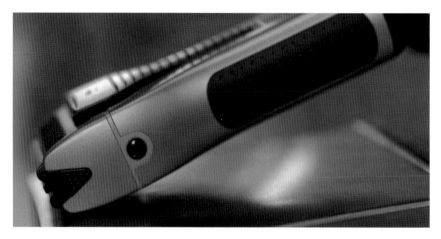

head. Foil heads are made of blades covered by one or more flexible metal foils that move back and forth. The heads have to be replaced fairly often. You move the shaver up and down on your face. Rotary heads, on the other hand, are made of circular cutters that rotate behind round combs. The heads can last up to several years without replacement. You move the shaver in a circular motion over the surface of your face.

There is no doubt that one—if not the only—advantage of electric shaving is that you can use the razor almost anywhere. The reality, however, is that no matter how you cut it, you'll never ever get as close a shave with an electric razor as you do with a traditional wet razor. But if you're in a situation where you have absolutely no alternative, there are a couple of things to keep in mind.

First, you should opt for a wet/dry electric razor, which is actually battery operated. The advantage of the electric wet/dry over the regular electric is that you use water and lather in combination with the shaver, thus providing your skin with some of the benefits of wet shaving. Second, shave after a shower, when your pores are clean and open. Third, use a badger-hair shaving brush and a high-quality lathering shaving cream or soap.

Another thing to remember is to apply alum block as a preshave on your face and neck to stiffen up your whiskers (see pages 54–55). Unlike traditional wet razors, electric shavers work better on dry hair when the hair shaft stands up on the face. And if there are certain parts of your face and neck that are more sensitive than others, shave those first, before the razor's head heats up and aggravates the skin further. Always keep your shaver clean, clearing the heads or comb slots of loose whiskers at least once week. And finally, if you can avoid using an electric shaver at all, please do.

SHAVING BRUSHES

We believe that the shaving brush is, in fact, one of the most important tools of shaving. The shaving brush was invented by the French in the eighteenth century, and until recently almost every man who shaved used one. But with modernization, with quick-and-easy disposable products like shaving foams, the use of a shaving brush quickly became a lost art. It's only with hindsight that men are finally starting to realize the importance of shaving, of taking care of their skin, and thus of the brush. We're convinced—and you will be too—that once you use a shaving brush, you'll never go back to fingers. You'll also find that using a brush is as efficient, if not more so, than not using one. You need a smaller amount of shaving cream for a rich and warm lather, and there's less waste.

Before brushes, there were sea sponges: men used them to lather up soap on their faces. The more traditional brush as we know it today (not the sponge kind but the bristle kind) was first introduced by the French in the 1750s. Since then, different kinds of bristles have been used—both natural and synthetic. But by far the best available brush today is made with badger hair.

The purpose of the brush is fourfold: it generates a rich and warm lather; it softens and lifts the beard off the face; it brings the right amount of warm water to the skin during the shaving process to open the pores and to lubricate the skin; and it gently exfoliates the surface of the skin to rid it of dead cells (see "The Actual Shave," page 82). By virtue of its numerous bristles, a shaving brush is the best way to generate a warm and unctuous lather. Think of it in terms of using a bath or shower gel and trying to generate lather with your fingers as opposed to with a sponge or washcloth. Clearly, you'll get better results with the latter, and while using less product. Rich lather is important because it protects and lubricates the skin. In addition, the gentle friction of the bristles on your face as you lather up warms the shaving cream and your skin, softening the beard and opening pores. The brush helps guide the direction of your whiskers as they loosen up in their pores, preparing them for the blade. The shaving brush is also ideal for ensuring adequate moisture to the face when shaving (see "Water," page 77): it captures and transports the moisture from the sink to your skin and beard. This is a far more efficient method of wetting your skin than cupping warm water in your hands and bringing it to your face when shaving, which is what you have to do without a brush. Finally, the brush provides gentle exfoliation and removes dead surface cells, something that fingers alone cannot do.

Like razor handles, shaving brushes are meant to be balanced, to fit comfortably in your hand, and to have a solid grip. Brush manufacturers usually offer different sizes and weights, depending on the size of your hand, and different types of bristles. The best bristle, however, is badger hair. Unlike boar's hair, horse's hair, or synthetic fibers, badger hair is naturally soft. It's the only hair type that retains water like a sponge. And with a small amount of cream, it gen-

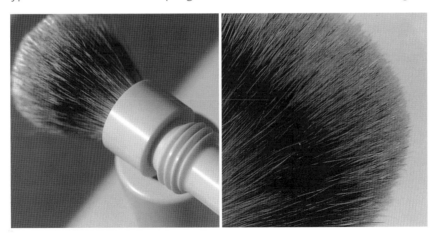

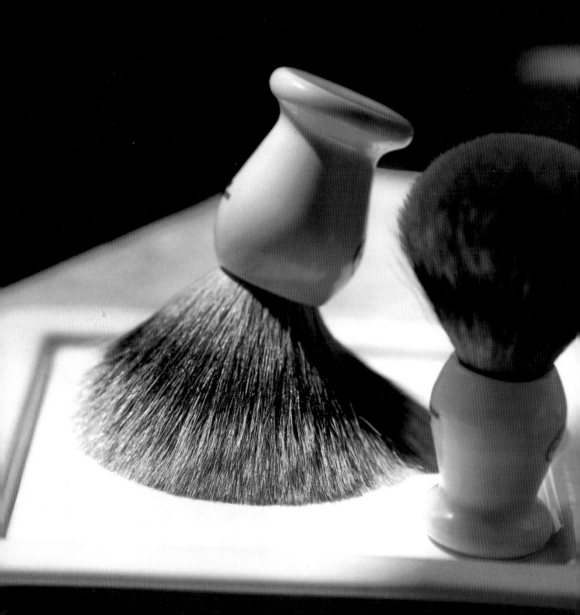

erates a very rich lather. Boar's and horse's hair, on the other hand, are coarse, which is uncomfortable for the skin, and they don't retain water. The best brushes are also those that are handcrafted, as they tend to keep their bristles, (and thus last) longer than machine-made ones.

There are essentially four different grades of badger hair: pure, fine, Silvertip, and High Mountain. The main differences between them are in hair quality (softness), density, and duration. High Mountain is the best and the most expensive—an average High Mountain badger brush can last ten years or more, whereas a pure badger lasts on average one to three years.

To care for your badger brush, it's important to rinse it well after each use, to flick it into the sink to remove excess water, and to hang it on a stand with the bristles facing down. This ensures that it's kept away from moisture and mildew, which softens the glue that holds the bristles to the handle, causing them to fall off. You'll know it's time to replace your brush when the bristles fall out or start to disintegrate in the water.

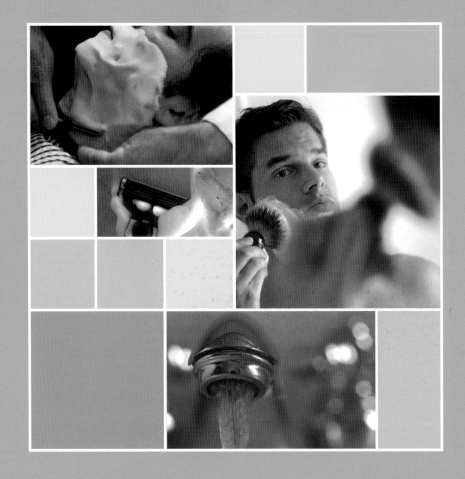

5 THE TECHNIQUES OF SHAVING

On average, men shave 5.33 times a week. That's about 21,000 shaves in a lifetime. For some, shaving has become such a routine that they can practically do it with their eyes closed, while eating breakfast or even behind the wheel. Unfortunately, many of these men have also acquired bad habits. Or they were simply never taught how to shave properly in the first place. They end up with bad results or injuries like razor burn, ingrown hairs, and nicks and cuts.

There's absolutely no reason why shaving should be a nasty experience. In fact, once the right tools and products have been selected, the only thing that stands between you and an ultrasmooth, close, comfortable, and injury-free shave is learning the proper techniques, which takes only a few moments. And since you'll be spending at least 3,500 hours of your adult life exercising these techniques, taking the time to learn them is probably the best investment you could ever make. Who knows, you might even enjoy it.

ELECTRIC SHAVING

The majority of men who shave prefer the wet shave (78 percent) to the electric. When done properly, wet shaving will give you the best possible results with no discomfort whatsoever. So why—you might rightfully ask—do other techniques exist at all? Most men who use electric razors choose it by default. (Although some men opt for electric razors for purely religious reasons: certain orthodox religions prohibit the use of a blade on or around the face.) They admit to having had a bad experience with wet shaving, and see electric razors as the only alternative. Others simply prefer the electric razor because it's supposedly less time-consuming. In fact, they're wrong on both counts.

Shaving injuries are *not* a direct result of wet shaving but of poor product and accessory selection, as well as poor technique. And electric shaving takes just as much time as wet shaving. The reason is simple: you never get as close a shave with electric shaving as you do with wet shaving, so you end up shaving twice or three times as much during the course of a day. (Electric razors are designed in such a way that the revolving blades are "screened-off" from the skin; if they don't get too close to the skin's surface, they won't catch and scrape it. The trade-off is that the blades never get close enough to the whiskers' base, which is why the shave is never superclose. Electric shavers can also contribute to ingrown hair problems: The blades sometimes rotate the hairs onto themselves and back toward the skin. After a while, the hair is "coerced" into growing inward instead of out, planting the seed for developing ingrown hairs.

Nevertheless, if you happen to be traveling somewhere where there's no fresh or running water to be found, using an electric razor is a second option. The first option, of course, is to just grow out your beard. There's no harm in playing the castaway every once in a while and giving your face and skin a chance to recuperate. But when using an electric razor, try rubbing a moistened alum block (see pages 54–55) over your face to soften the beard and to remove the excess oil.

THE ART OF WET SHAVING

Wet shaving makes the shave as smooth, close, and comfortable as possible. With the right choice of products and accessories—as well as proper habits— you can greatly reduce your chances of injury, if not eliminate them altogether.

Traditional wet shaving has been around since prehistoric times. Wet shaving involves the use of a shaving brush, shaving soap or cream, water, a blade, and a razor. The fundamental principles of wet shaving revolve around the importance of hot water, a rich and warm lather, and the actual techniques themselves.

WATER

Even before the discovery of soap, men used water to shave. Hot water, in particular, has always been an extremely important element in the art of shaving. Its purpose is to prepare and cleanse the skin, to provide moisture for the lathering process, to ensure that the skin is sufficiently hydrated when shaving, and to soften the beard. (Note the use of the word *hot,* as in "hot but not scalding.")

Actually, wetting and maintaining the hair wet throughout the shaving

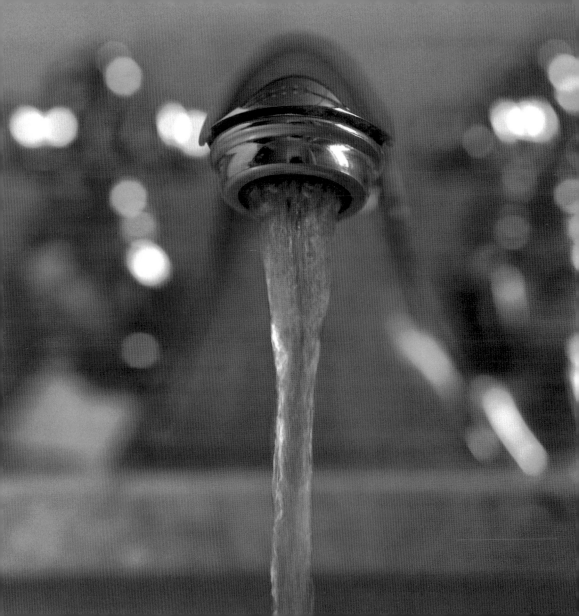

process is key for two reasons: it lubricates the skin and it opens the pores. The water's ability to lubricate the skin ensures that the razor and blade will glide smoothly over the surface being shaved, and that the skin will be less dry and scratchy after the shave. Furthermore, the water's heat dilates the blood vessels on the skin's surface, which in turn opens and relaxes pores. When a pore is relaxed, the hair follicle in it becomes loose and pliable, and far more manageable. With a soft and manageable beard, whiskers can be guided easily in one direction or another with a shaving brush or fingers. The blade is then at a better angle to catch the hair without catching the skin.

Cold water constricts blood vessels, tightens pores, and makes hair follicles stiff. When whiskers are stiff, the beard is resistant, which makes it harder for the blade to catch each hair. In fact, because hot water plays such an integral role in the

WATER AND HAIR

Human hair is made up in most part of keratin, a highly complex protein that's not soluble in water but capable of absorbing water and oil. When the hair is wet, its elasticity increases by about 90 percent, and it loses about 60 percent of its strength. Since discomfort in shaving is often associated with pulling the hair—that is, the resistance of the hair shaft to the cutting edge— it is obvious why the hair needs to be wet; it will give less resistance to the blade, and the shave will thus be more comfortable.

art of wet shaving, we strongly recommend that you shave during or right after a hot shower, when your pores are relaxed and your beard softened. And *never* shave before a shower or when your skin is dry, not well prepared, and taut. If you don't want to shower before shaving, splash water on your face and neck, or use a wet hot towel as traditional barbershops do. Rest it on your face and

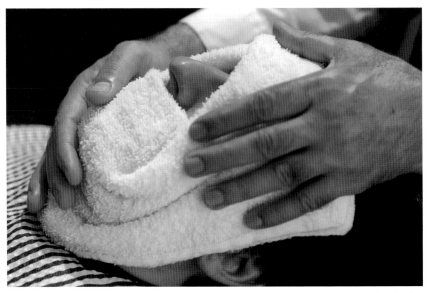

neck for about half a minute, or enough time for your skin to take in both the heat and the moisture.

To start the shaving process, you need to generate a rich and warm lather. Hot water, for that reason, is essential, because it's the medium by which a shaving brush lathers up traditional shaving soap in a dish or bowl, or by which a brush or fingers lather up shaving cream directly onto the face (see "The Products of Shaving," page 00). We strongly recommend, however, that you use a badger-hair shaving brush, because a brush is the most efficient way of wetting your hair and your skin and keeping them wet during the process.

On the other hand, splashing *cold* water on your face and neck after a shave is highly recommended: it gets rid of shaving cream residue, closes the pores, regenerates, and refreshes.

PRESHAVE PREPARATION

Determining the Grain

Before you even *think* of picking up your razor or turning on the tap, look in the mirror. Examine your face closely—no, not for its devastating good looks but to discover the direction in which the hair on your face grows, which is called the *grain*. For most men, whiskers on their faces grow down. Check to see whether the hair on your neck grows in the same direction as the hair on your face. If it doesn't, make sure you adjust accordingly to shave with the grain. (The direction of the grain stays consistent throughout your shaving career, so you only need to figure this out once.)

It's important to determine the grain because after lathering up, you have to shave *with* the grain—that is, in the direction of growth. Shaving with the grain first removes approximately 80 percent of the hair's length. Shaving *against* the grain first can cause razor burn, skin irritations, and ingrown hairs (see "The Injuries of Shaving," page 97). If you want a closer shave, or if your beard is extra thick and tough, then and *only* then should you relather and shave either against or across the grain. After the first shave, the hair shaft is shorter and the risk of the hair folding back onto itself and into the skin is greatly reduced.

Applying Preshave Oil

The purpose of applying preshave oil is to provide a protective barrier between your skin and the sharpness of the blade. It's particularly recommended for men with sensitive skin, tough beards, ingrown hairs, and razor burn. High-quality preshave oils do not leave any oily residue on the skin. They're automatically wiped off when the blade glides over the skin. Look for preshave oils that contain natural essential oils with warming properties to open pores and soften the beard, making it even more manageable. Before shaving, rub a small amount of preshave oil in the palm of your hands (a nickel-size amount should do) and massage it into your wet beard. Use upward motions to lift the beard off the face. Before shaving, wash your hands to remove oily residue.

THE ACTUAL SHAVE

Lather Up

The lathering process—either with fingers or preferably a brush—is crucial because it serves multiple purposes: lubricating the skin, protecting it, directly softening the beard, and making the whiskers more manageable. Lather is an effective buffer between the blade and the skin. This additional protective layer ensures a comfortable shave. It also ensures that the blade glides smoothly over the surface being shaved.

To obtain the richest lather possible, use a traditional high-fat-content shaving soap or shaving cream with a high-quality badger-hair shaving brush. When

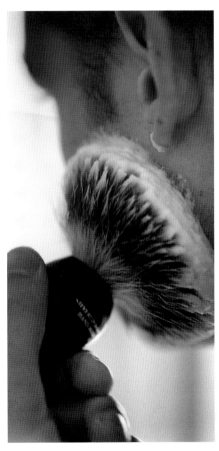

properly whisked, the lather generated from shaving soap or creams and brush is by far the most unctuous. The richer the lather, the more the skin is protected, and the more comfortable and close the shave. Continuing the lathering process on the face and neck with a shaving brush, as opposed to just using fingers, has additional advantages: the brush's bristles gently exfoliate and warm the skin, open the pores, warm up the lather, and soften the beard. The additional heat opens pores further and makes whiskers even more pliable. The bristles also help raise the whiskers to facilitate the contact of the blade with the hair follicles.

Fill the sink with hot water, dip the brush in it for about fifteen seconds, and then remove it; alternatively, hold the brush under a hot running faucet. Do not tap excess water off the brush. The point is for the bristles to retain as much water as possible so it can keep your face hydrated and protected during the shaving process. With circular motions, run the bristles over the soap to generate lather. The longer you whisk, the richer the lather, and the more protection it provides the skin. Fifteen seconds should do.

If you're using a lathering cream instead of soap, wet the tip of the shaving brush slightly, open the center of the brush, and place two fingertips' worth of cream into the center of the brush. Close up the tip and submerge it in hot water for about twenty seconds. Remove from the water and begin lathering. If you feel you need more water during the course of shaving, dip the tip of the brush in water and flick it gently to removing excess, if necessary.

Once the brush is on your face, it's important to use just the right amount of pressure. Too much can cause bristles to flatten on your face, which flattens whiskers; too little won't provide enough friction for good lather.

Shaving Strokes

Dip the blade in hot water and start shaving. The blade should be hot to ease the cutting; just think of it in terms of a hot blade cutting through butter. And remember to shave *with* the grain first (see above, "Determining the Grain").

Men shave with different styles, starting on different parts of the face. But if you're trying to break bad habits and to acquire healthy new ones, the following techniques work best. First, use your finger to remove a small amount of lather next to your sideburns to determine where they start and end. Align the blade with the end of the sideburn and start shaving downward (with the grain), applying little pressure on the handle. Use a steady, consistent motion.

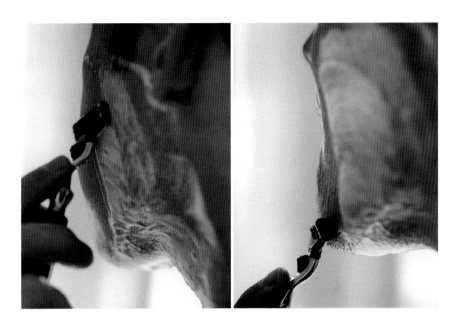

Too much pressure on the handle will irritate the skin by removing too many surface cells, and it won't yield a closer shave anyway. Pay close attention— many irritations and razor burns are a result of excessive pressure.

Razor strokes should be neither too long nor too short. Like most things in life, they should be just right. On cheeks and throat, about two inches is a good length. In the mustache area below the nose, one downward stroke is usually sufficient. You want to draw an imaginary line along your jawline, separating the face from the neck. Shave the jawline with small strokes above the line, then small strokes below it. Don't attempt to go around the curve of the chin in one fell swoop, because you'll get nicked. Always remember to adjust the direction of your strokes on the neck and lower neck area according to the direction of the grain.

Thoroughly rinse your razor with warm water to remove excess hair, dirt, and lather between strokes. Since the water in the sink might get soapy from the lathering process, hot water directly from the tap is best.

For an even closer shave, relather your face and neck. Shave against the grain using extra-gentle strokes, starting from the bottom of the neck area and working your way up to the cheeks, the mustache area under your nose, and the chin. "The Challenges of Shaving" (page 89) contains special instructions—how to shave around goatees or mustaches, for example.

AFTERSHAVE CARE

Thoroughly rinse your face and neck with cold water to tighten pores, to invigorate, and to refresh. Pat skin dry. In the event of a cut or nick, immediately apply an antiseptic styptic pencil or moistened alum block to help stop bleeding. (For more information on styptic pencils and alum blocks, see "The Products of Shaving," pages 54–55.)

Whenever you shave, a thin layer of skin gets removed, leaving what's underneath sensitive and dry. Therefore, it's important to apply an alcohol- and fragrance-free aftershave balm or gel to soothe, nourish, moisturize, and disin-

SHAVING TECHNIQUES AT A GLANCE

- Always shave after or during a hot shower, never before.
- Always use hot water while shaving. Hot water cleanses the skin, softens the beard, and opens pores.
- Before shaving, apply preshave oil to protect the skin and to further open pores.
- Use a high-quality badger shaving brush and traditional shaving cream or soap to generate the richest lather possible.
- Always shave with the grain first. If you need an even closer shave, relather and shave against or across the grain.
- Avoid applying too much pressure on the razor's handle. Excessive pressure causes razor burn and skin irritations and doesn't give you a closer shave.
- For nicks, cuts, or razor burn, immediately apply a styptic pencil or moistened alum block to disinfect and help stop bleeding.
- After shaving, apply an aftershave balm or gel to nourish, soothe, and moisturize the skin. Certain gels and balms also help maintain healthy skin and promote skin-tissue regeneration in between shaves.

fect the skin, to help regenerate cell growth, and to help maintain healthy skin (see "The Products of Shaving," pages 49–54). Gently pat the product on the skin; don't rub it in. Rubbing will irritate the skin. Allow the gel or balm to air-dry naturally. If you use alcohol-based cologne, don't apply it directly to the shaved area—you want to keep alcohol away from your face as much as possible. Instead, dab it on the back of your neck, lower neck, or shoulders for the same sensational effect.

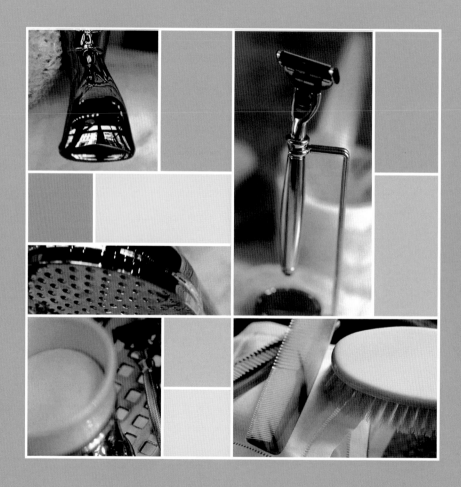

6 THE CHALLENGES OF SHAVING

To shave or not to shave? *That* is the question. Over the years, whiskers have taken on all sorts of shapes and sizes, catering to fashionable, political, religious, personal, and even economic views. Full beards, collar beards, mustaches, goatees, sideburns, clean-shaven faces: all evoke a distinctive look and personality. And for each, it takes skill and finesse to achieve the proper look.

BASIC TECHNIQUES AND MAINTENANCE
FOR BEARDS, MUSTACHES, GOATEES, AND MORE

If what you're going for is a totally new look—by changing the shape of your beard or growing one in—there are a couple of things you need to know. First, be aware that it will alter your profile and the shape of your face. Second, it takes on average one week to a month—depending on how fast your beard grows and how thick it is—to achieve a full look. After about two weeks (earlier

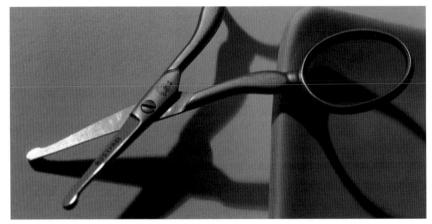

for a goatee or small mustache), you can start outlining certain parts of your face and separating the neckline with a razor or an "outliner" (a trimmer specially made to trim the beard's extremities). After that, you can start using a professional clipper, a trimmer, or sharp scissors and comb to create an even length. Touch up the extremities with a mustache razor—a double-sided razor with one side much smaller than the other. The small side is for getting into those hard-to-reach areas, like around the lip, over the chin, and under the nose. We recommend that you get a professional barber trim every month to properly reshape your whiskers.

Once you've achieved the look you want, you need to maintain it, of course. Like the hair on your head, your beard should be shampooed and conditioned on a regular basis; in fact, every time you shampoo and condition your hair in the shower, you should do the same for your beard. Always pat dry and moisturize your beard and face, and apply aftershave balm or gel after showering. This will make your beard soft and get rid of any flakiness or itchy feeling. Then use a small mustache or beard comb (or a regular comb with small, narrow teeth) to comb your whiskers down, in the direction of the grain. To hold your whiskers in place all day, touch up with a mustache wax for a clean, well-groomed look.

If you're entirely shaving off a beard or mustache, first trim it as short as you can with scissors or with a professional trimmer to remove as much hair as possible, then shave off the rest with a razor. This will make it easier for you to monitor the shaving strokes and to prevent excess hair from clogging and dulling the blade. Your newly exposed skin (the part that was previously covered by facial hair) will be unusually sensitive to cold and sunlight, so be sure to protect it.

BEARDS

The beard was at one time considered the lazy man's fashion. In fact, many men still grow out their beards because they just don't want to be bothered with shaving and hate the whole concept, or because at some point they had a painful experience. But the reality is that a beard, like any other whisker style, warrants a certain amount of maintenance and effort. First, you need to choose the style. Beard length and rate of whisker growth set the pace for how often it needs to be trimmed. If the beard grows quickly and the style is short, then count on tending to your beard three or four times a week. If the style is long, then the beard needs tending every ten days to two weeks.

Also, remember that when you have a beard, there's nothing more unattractive than an unshaven neck or scraggly beard. So the areas surrounding the beard—the ones that define the beard—should be kept up and clean-shaven, as though you had no beard at all. Keep trimming scissors close at hand, and treat yourself to a professional trim every once in a while to assure that your whiskers are properly outlined. There's nothing like a well-trained, objective hand to give you perspective and self-assurance.

MUSTACHES

From the short, under-the-nose strip to a long and lanky "handlebar," the mustache makes a huge statement. The trademark of men of elegance and power, mustaches have been around for as long as there have been men of fashion. The mustache style is determined by the length of its corners and how far it extends from the lips to the outer reaches of the face and beyond. To determine what look suits you best, check out the distance between the bottom of your nose and your upper lip. The greater the distance, the fuller the mustache should be. Use an electric outliner or scissors to trim the upper lip. Also remember to have your mustache trimmed every time you go in for a haircut or for a professional shave.

GOATEES

The goatee, a style that covers the mustache area and chin, has multiple personalities. Long and droopy, it can look very Fu Manchu; short and trim, it can give off slightly menacing airs.

Like a beard, a goatee can be worn at different lengths, but it needs to be carefully maintained around the edges. The exterior edge should be shaved from the outside of the face toward the goatee, in a horizontal direction—*never* use vertical strokes. The inside line under the lower lip should be left alone; if necessary, use a small mustache trimmer. In general, goatees tend to look good on men with short hair and shaved heads.

SIDEBURNS

Sideburns are an important part of every hairstyle. Their length can totally change your look. Whatever their shape or length, make sure the tips (or lengths) on both sides are always even and of equal thickness. Look straight into the mirror when you shave your cheeks, right below your sideburns. Accidents happen when you shave one side of your face while looking straight into the mirror, then completely turn your head to shave the other, thus losing sight of the first. Also, switch hands when you shave each side of your face. Keeping the razor in the same hand for shaving both sides usually results in asymmetrical sideburns. Your barber or hairstylist will give you a little trim to maintain thickness whenever you go in.

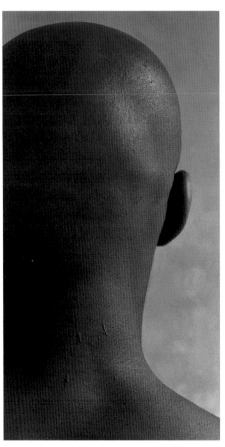

HEAD

The head shave has become very popular in recent years, and the rules for shaving the head are the same as those for the face: opening the pores, lathering, shaving with the grain, relathering, and shaving across or against the grain. Keep in mind that some areas might be more sensitive than others. One in particular extends from the back of the head to the neck, so avoid shaving against the grain in that spot. Another tricky part is right behind the ears: gently pull the ear forward and shave behind it with a downward stroke. Gliding your fingers on your head along with the razor will also help you catch any spots that you can't see. The very first time you shave your head, cut off as much hair as possible before using the razor. And take it slowly.

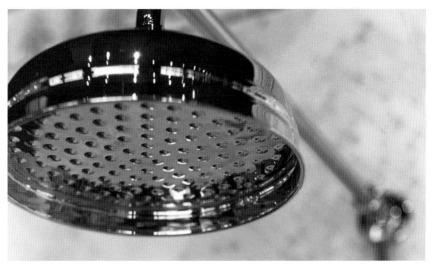

SHAVING IN THE SHOWER

Many men swear by shaving in the shower and wouldn't do it any other way. It saves time, since you're in the shower anyway. And the continuous stream of hot water and steam helps to soften the beard and keep the skin hydrated. And cleaning up and rinsing off are a whole lot easier. The one frustration is that the mirror tends to fog up, making it difficult to see. So lather up some soap in your hands and cover the mirror with it. After about five seconds, remove the suds by splashing hot water on the mirror (don't use your hands or a towel). The mirror will stay fog-free for about ten minutes.

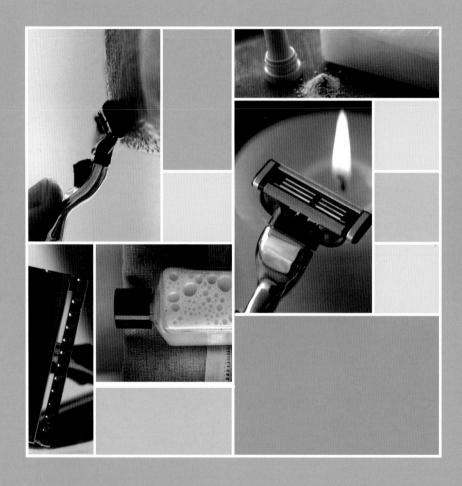

7 THE INJURIES OF SHAVING

There's nothing worse than a painful shave, except maybe the unfortunate *aftermath* of a painful shave—ingrown hairs and razor bumps, razor burn, and nicks and cuts. Ouch! And it's probably one of the reasons why some men decide to stop shaving altogether and to grow a beard. The irony of it all is that there's really no reason for anyone to suffer any of these injuries in the first place. If you use the proper tools, products, and techniques, your shave should be smooth and superclose, as well as pain- and injury-free. If you're dealing with residual injuries from bygone days (before you had a chance to read this book, of course, and discover the wonderful world of painless shaving), then you need to address them immediately.

There are essentially three different types of shaving injuries: ingrown hairs and razor bumps, razor burn, and nicks and cuts.

INGROWN HAIRS

WHAT ARE INGROWN HAIRS?

An ingrown hair is created when a hair is either pushed back into the skin while shaving or somehow prevented from growing out of it, or when the hair curls back onto itself and reenters the same follicle. In both cases, the body's natural reaction is to treat the "intruding" hair like a foreign body. And when any foreign matter penetrates the skin, the skin gets inflamed and infected. Ingrown hairs can also occur when skin is so dry and tight that the skin itself acts as a barrier to the hair's growth, and the hair gets stuck in its own follicle and continues to grow underneath the skin. Sebum, the natural oily secretion of the skin's sebaceous glands, then starts to accumulate in the closed pore and surrounds the ingrown hair, forming an unsightly and infected pimple. If the hair doesn't come out within a few days, the accumulation of sebum causes a cystlike mass in the follicle, which traps the hair even more by anchoring it deep into the skin.

WHO GETS INGROWN HAIRS?

Basically, all skin types are susceptible, although certain men are more prone than others: men with curly hair or dry skin, for example; curly hair has a natural tendency to curl back onto itself and get caught in the skin. Men who are of African American or of southern Mediterranean descent (or any men who have dark skin) seem to be more prone to developing ingrown hair and razor bumps, which are essentially an aggravated case of ingrown hairs. And dry skin can create an impenetrable barrier underneath which the hair gets stuck.

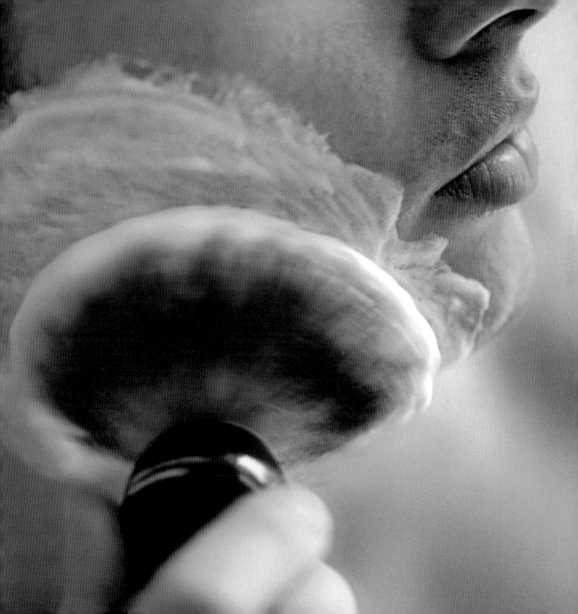

WHAT CAUSES INGROWN HAIRS?

Poor Products

Lack of proper facial protection is one of the main culprits behind ingrown hairs. Most products on the market do not offer adequate protection, and they do not soften the beard enough to make the hairs pliable. The ones you select should provide the extra layer that you need between your skin and the blade (see page 37). Also, since dry skin can contribute to the problem, stay away from shaving foams and gels, aftershaves, and other shaving products containing alcohol, synthetic perfumes, dyes, and numbing agents (menthol and benzocaine) that will dry out your skin. Avoid those containing alcohol or numbing agents that tighten pores: these include shaving foams, gels, and poor-quality shaving soaps and creams, as well as astringents, alcohol-based aftershaves, perfumes, and colognes. Don't use any products that are cold when dispensed, such as foams or gels. In reaction to the cold, pores tighten, the beard becomes stiff, and the hairs can easily get stuck under the skin.

Poor Techniques

It's very important to shave *with* the grain (see "The Techniques of Shaving," pages 81–85). Shaving *against* the grain the first time around can push the hair back into its pore. Only after you've completed your first round and lathered up again can you shave against or across the grain. The second time around, the hair is much shorter and is not likely to be pushed back into the skin. (Remember that the direction of the grain can be different on your neck and face.) And

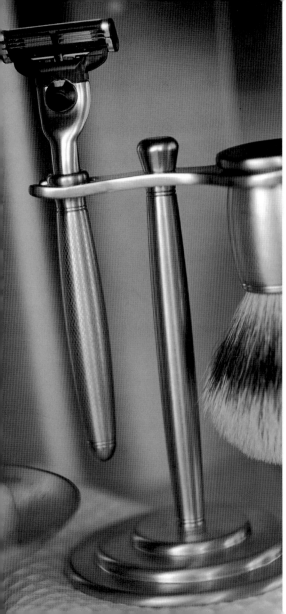

always use a light stroke. Too much pressure on the skin can exacerbate an existing ingrown hair by injuring and infecting it again. Use protective preshave oil to provide a layer between the blade and skin to prevent ingrown hairs, or to help the blade glide over whatever bumps or ingrown hairs you already have.

Poor Tools

A dull and dirty blade is another culprit. It won't necessarily *cause* an ingrown hair, but it will *aggravate* whatever ingrown hair might be there. A dull blade will exert more resistance when cutting the hair than a sharp one, and each time a germ-infected blade scrapes over an ingrown hair, it can reinfect it. An aggravated ingrown hair eventually turns into a razor bump, which is even more difficult to get rid of. Razor bumps can also leave scars when (and if) they heal. So make sure that you thoroughly clean, rinse, and dry your blade after each use. An accumulation of bacteria—from a dirty blade to a rusty one—is not something that you ever want near your face. Store your razor in a clean and dry place, away from moisture, preferably on a stand so that the blade is not in contact with anything. Change your blade on a regular basis and certainly at the first sign of dullness or discomfort. Depending on the thickness of your beard, we recommend that you put a new one in every three to five shaves. We also recommend that you use a good-quality badger-hair brush. The brush naturally lifts the beard off the face and softens it, thereby reducing the chances of developing ingrown hairs. The shaving brush also exfoliates dead skin, thereby softening the skin, making it easier for the hair to grow naturally.

HOW DO YOU TREAT INGROWN HAIRS?

If you use the right products and techniques, you won't get ingrown hairs in the first place. But there are products on the market that claim to heal them. Most of them contain alcohol and salicylic acid. The alcohol is meant to disinfect and the salicylic acid to peel off the external layer of skin. Peeling and drying out is only temporary relief; the fact is that the hair is still stuck in the skin. What ends up happening is that the acid and alcohol tighten the pore even more, constricting the ingrown hair, making matters worse.

We recommend an entirely different approach. First, treat the hair with a natural disinfectant like lavender essential oil or tea tree oil to reduce the inflammation and redness. Then, instead of drying up and peeling off the ingrown hair, try "maturing" it instead to speed up the ingrown hair's life span and to get to the healing part faster. Use shea butter, a natural moisturizer and anti-inflammatory. At bedtime, apply a small amount directly on the ingrown hair, and leave it on overnight. Shea butter eventually coaxes the ingrown hair out of its follicle. You can also use olive, jojoba, hazelnut, or almond oil. It's important to use a good aftershave balm or cream, applied after each shave and at bedtime to help healing. Look for ones that contain a natural disinfectant, like red algae, to avoid the risk of future infections. Finally, avoid wearing tight-collared shirts that the ingrown hairs would come in contact with. The friction of the fabric can increase the chances of developing or worsening ingrown hairs. The use of a gentle exfoliant twice a week is also a good idea.

RAZOR BURN

WHAT IS RAZOR BURN?

Razor burn is the result of removing too much skin while shaving. It can be so painful that men have sworn off shaving for years. It's like a bad scrape all over your face, and it leaves your skin red, burning, and irritated.

WHO GETS RAZOR BURN?

Razor burn is a problem that can affect all skin types, targeting in particular men with sensitive skin and fair complexions (see page 25). And it's a problem that can be very easily avoided with a few minor adjustments.

WHAT CAUSES RAZOR BURN?

As with ingrown hairs, the cause is not shaving itself but poor technique and products.

Poor Techniques

Excessive blade pressure on the face and shaving against the grain the first time around contribute to razor burn. Many men think that if they apply lots of pressure, they'll get closer results. In fact, what they end up with is raw skin. Excessive pressure will cause the blade to scrape off too many layers of skin, causing severe burning, irritation, and redness. Always pay close attention to the amount of pressure you apply with the razor. The blade should practically hover over the skin, catching only hairs and nothing else.

Shaving against the grain the first time around can also contribute to razor burn. When you shave against the grain, the blade encounters a lot of resistance from stiff whiskers. To counteract the resistance, the natural tendency is to apply more pressure and to repeat the shaving stroke over the same area. But this will unnecessarily strip the skin of some of its layers.

Poor Tools and Products

Avoid throwaway or disposable razors, especially single-blade, which are far less efficient than two- or three-blade razors simply because they have only one blade and are usually made with lesser-quality steel. As a result, you'll be tempted to shave over the same area more than once, unnecessarily removing a layer of skin each time.

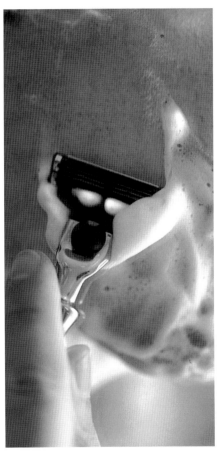

Poor products can also cause razor burn. Shaving foams or gels, or products used without water, are inherently bad because they just don't provide enough protection for the skin during the shaving process. And anything that contains numbing agents (see "The Products of Shaving," page 47) can affect your awareness of blade pressure on your face. Use shaving soaps or creams that are high in fat and moisture so they provide your skin with the protection and lubrication it needs during the shaving process. Avoid products that contain dyes, synthetic fragrances, and alcohol, all of which can irritate and dry out skin and cause allergic reactions. Add extra protection to your skin by applying preshave oil. The oil coats the skin so that the blade simply glides over it, cutting only hairs and protecting external skin layers. We also recommend that you use a badger-hair shaving brush so that a maximum amount of moisture is brought to the skin when you lather up and shave. And use an alcohol-, fragrance-, and dye-free moisturizing aftershave to naturally soothe and disinfect the skin in between shaves. A moisturizing aftershave has the added advantage of helping skin tissue regenerate and heal in time for the next shave.

HOW DO YOU TREAT RAZOR BURN?

If the damage has been done and you have burn, you can alleviate the unpleasant sensation by applying a cold compress or cold water mixed with a few drops of vitamin E, lavender, chamomile, or calendula essential oil to your face. Splashing rose water on your face also helps. Known for their soothing and healing properties, these essential oils will reduce redness and irritation on the skin's surface. You can also apply alum block (see pages 54–55) to help relieve razor burn, although it may sting a bit. Simply moisten the block with cold water and gently rub it over your face. After a few seconds, splash water over your entire face to remove any alum-block residue. Then apply a facial moisturizer or moisturizing aftershave balm that contains natural ingredients such as red algae and shea butter. These ingredients have inherent healing, anti-inflammatory, and cell-regenerative properties and help maintain healthy skin. Dab or gently pat the moisturizer on; don't rub or massage it into the skin because this can cause further burning. Finally, it's very important to apply a moisturizer to your face and neck to help heal and regenerate the skin in between shaves.

NICKS AND CUTS

WHAT ARE NICKS AND CUTS?

Nicks and cuts are slices in the skin that draw blood. Whether you're a seasoned shaver or a new member, nicks and cuts are one of those unfortunate facts of life that you just have to deal with. So the best way to avoid them is to anticipate them.

WHO GETS GETS NICKS AND CUTS AND WHAT CAUSES THEM?

Inattentive shavers. The number one cause for nicks and cuts is lack of attention. You stayed up too late the night before, the phone is ringing off the hook, you're late for work. Or you're at a friend's house, and there's no mirror in the bathroom, but you figure you know your face so well that you can shave without one. The next thing you know, your razor slips, you lose your concentration, you miscalculate the curve of your jawline, and wham!

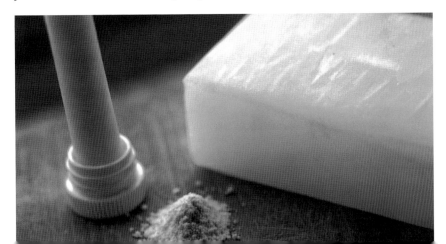

In addition to inattentiveness, the primary culprits are disposable razors that don't swivel. These stiff razors make it hard to accurately follow the contours of the face and to monitor pressure. So use a razor that has a swiveling head and a well-balanced handle.

HOW DO YOU TREAT NICKS AND CUTS?

The first thing you need to do is to stop the bleeding, then to disinfect the cut. Moisten the tip of a styptic pencil or an alum block with cold water and apply it directly to the cut for about five seconds, or until the bleeding stops. The styptic pencil or alum block disinfects and speeds up the healing process by constricting blood vessels and closing up the cut. Once the cut is closed, apply an alcohol-, fragrance-, and dye-free moisturizing aftershave to the face. Make sure you dab it on, instead of massaging or rubbing it in, so as not to reopen the cut. To minimize the chances of future nicks and cuts, sufficiently lubricate and protect your skin before, and during, the shaving process. Use preshave oil and a rich, lathering shaving cream. And, as always, make sure your blade is sharp and clean.

Now you've read the worst of it. Perhaps you drew blood, but you definitely survived. And, more important, you looked into the enemy's eyes and saw victory. Yours. So put those fears behind you, and bid farewell to the days of painful shaving. *Adiós* to ingrown hairs, razor burn, and nicks and cuts. It's time to start anew.

ACKNOWLEDGMENTS

Many thanks to Catherine Bardey for her invaluable work on the text; without you, this book would not have been possible. Also thanks to Susan Salinger for the beautiful photography; our agent Dean Williamson; Chris Pavone, Caitlin Daniels Israel, Mark McCauslin, Alison Forner, Andrea Rosen, and everyone else at Clarkson Potter; Nathalie and Gaby Monteriano; Elize Gambard; Michael Felton; Boris Mirzankandov; Sam Mirzakan; Karina Negals; Manuel Borrego; Sonny Salomon; Urban Archaeology; the Gillette Company; and the residents of New York City.

INDEX

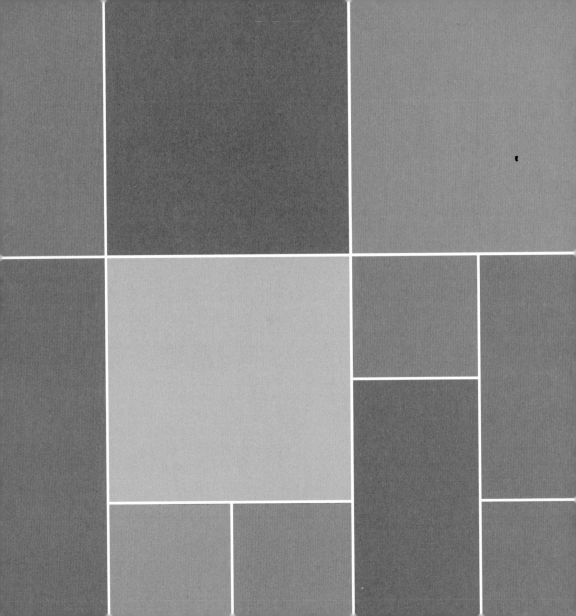